Your Child's Mental Health Diagnosis

Your Child's Mental Health Diagnosis

A Comprehensive and Compassionate Guide for Parents

Jacqueline Corcoran

ROWMAN & LITTLEFIELD
Lanham • Boulder • New York • London

Published by Rowman & Littlefield
An imprint of The Rowman & Littlefield Publishing Group, Inc.
4501 Forbes Boulevard, Suite 200, Lanham, Maryland 20706
www.rowman.com

86-90 Paul Street, London EC2A 4NE

British Library Cataloguing in Publication Information Available

Library of Congress Cataloging-in-Publication Data

Names: Corcoran, Jacqueline, author.
   Title: Your child's mental health diagnosis : a comprehensive and compassionate guide for parents / Jacqueline Corcoran.
   Description: Lanham : Rowman & Littlefield, [2024] | Includes bibliographical references and index. | Summary: "Your Child's Mental Health Diagnosis provides the most up-to-date information on mental disorders in children, delivered in a warm and supportive manner with many examples to which parents can relate. Each chapter covers symptoms, the diagnosing process, possible treatments to discuss with doctors, parenting your child, and self-care for parents"-- Provided by publisher.
   Identifiers: LCCN 2023048120 (print) | LCCN 2023048121 (ebook) | ISBN 9781538175033 (cloth) | ISBN 9781538175040 (epub)
   Subjects: LCSH: Child psychiatry. | Child mental health. | Child mental health--Evaluation.
   Classification: LCC RJ499 .C67 2024 (print) | LCC RJ499 (ebook) | DDC 618.92/89--dc23/eng/20240104
   LC record available at https://lccn.loc.gov/2023048120
   LC ebook record available at https://lccn.loc.gov/2023048121

Acknowledgments to the children, teens, and parents I have worked with throughout the years for deepening my capacity to understand diagnosis in youth and assist families in recovery. I hope to honor your lived experience by channeling it into guidance for other parents whose children are diagnosed with mental health disorders.

Contents

Acknowledgments

Thank you especially to Courtney Wolk Benjamin, my coauthor of *Child and Adolescent Mental Health in Social Work: A Casebook*, and also to Joseph Walsh, my coauthor of *Clinical Assessment and Diagnosis in Social Work Practice* and *Mental Health in Social Work: A Casebook on Diagnosis and Strengths-Based Assessment*. Both coauthors' clinical wisdom and professional and research knowledge have been invaluable to the background of this book.

Thank you also to Dawn Eichen, who contributed to the Eating Disorders chapter in *Child and Adolescent Mental Health in Social Work*, which informed chapter 5 in this book. Colleagues at the School of Social Policy and Practice, Kimberly McKay, Kaitlyn Regan, and Stephanie Chando, contributed reading recommendations for parents of LGBTQ youth. Finally, I'm grateful for the efforts of Miette Gourlay, Alex Kenner, and Dara Jih-Cook, who worked so hard to assist in the preparation of *Your Child's Mental Health Diagnosis: A Comprehensive and Compassionate Guide for Parents*.

Introduction

If you've picked up this book, it's likely your child has been diagnosed with a mental health disorder, you're a concerned relative, or you're wondering if your child shows signs of a mental disorder. You may feel alone and overwhelmed amid your child's struggles. It's heartbreaking when your child suffers. Most parents would rather bear pain themselves than see it in their children. At the same time, since you are your child's "safe" person—they know that you love them unconditionally and are not going anywhere—you are often the receptacle of their conflicts and frustration. This isn't easy to put up with either, especially after all you do for your child.

With these myriad feelings, you may feel isolated from "normal families." You see postings on social media and hear from friends and relatives about family members supposedly having fun together. Of course, we understand that social media may not represent reality fairly, but we often do not share these other experiences and feel alone.

You are *not* alone, as mental health disorders are increasing for children in the United States. According to the National Survey of Children's Health, one in six children, six to seventeen years old, is now diagnosed with a mental disorder.[1] This rate translates into 7.7 million children in the United States.

Your Child's Mental Health Diagnosis: A Comprehensive and Compassionate Guide for Parents is informed by my academic knowledge and clinical and parenting experiences with struggling children. This multifaceted level of expertise allows me to answer all the various questions that may run through your mind:

What is wrong with my child?

How is my child going to manage in life?

Did I do anything to cause what my child is going through?

What can I do now?

Does a diagnosis explain how my child feels and acts?

What diagnosis fits my child's pattern of reactions and behaviors?

Can we solve this without medication?

Does a diagnosis help my child get intervention?

What rights does my child have in school?

Will my child be able to take care of himself/herself when I'm no longer here?

Can my child be normal?

Can a diagnosis fix my child?

What caused this in my child?

What's the best way to parent this child?

What are the best-researched options for intervention? What do parents find most useful?

Where do I go to get help?

How can I pay for all this?

How can I maintain my own sanity amid the stress of having a child with an emotional or behavioral disorder?

You may have checked out this book because you're having difficulty navigating services. And no wonder you're confused—the US mental health system is very fragmented, with no single entry point for screening, assessment, and treatment. Instead, a dizzying array of systems, settings, players, and personnel are involved. *Your Child's Mental Health Diagnosis* will help you sort out the effective interventions available to your child and family.

If you're worried about your child's mental health, you undoubtedly suffer from stress, heartbreak, disappointment, worry, grief, frustration, and guilt. Although you love your children, you don't always like them, and taking care of them through the routines of daily living is stress-inducing. Did you do something to cause your child to be like this?

There is a long history of blaming mothers for various disorders. For example, in the 1960s, the dominant theory for autism was the cold, removed "refrigerator mother." Of course, at this stage, we know that parenting has nothing to do with the origins of autism. And, for all the disorders, a parent simply has to be "good enough." (We will talk more about what this means in subsequent chapters.) But parenting a child with mental disabilities takes more effort and a toll on your own mental health. For that reason, *Your Child's Mental Health Diagnosis* offers support and validation, and information informed by research evidence and my clinical expertise. In this book, chapters are organized by each of the disorders that are commonly diagnosed today. In each chapter, the criteria for the diagnosis are summarized so you understand the symptoms involved and their persistence. Frequently co-occurring disorders are also covered.

Of course, the big question parents often ask is *why*? Why does my child think, feel, and act in these ways? Causes will be discussed through a holistic consideration of psychological and social contributors, as well as biological influences. Subsequent sections answer other vital questions: Can my child be cured? If there is no cure, what is helpful for successful adjustment? What are the treatments that have received the most research backing? How do these dovetail with parents' experiences? Where can you find effective treatments? How will you pay for them? Should I give my child medication: the pros and cons to consider? What about your own mental health? How can you take care of yourself so your quality of life doesn't take a hit amid all you do for your child?

MENTAL DISORDER AND DIAGNOSIS

Before embarking on each disorder-specific chapter, here I will "draw back the curtain" on the diagnostic process in the United States, involving the American Psychiatric Association and the influence of pharmaceutical companies. This information does not diminish your or your child's suffering, but it does offer needed context for the "diagnostic enterprise" in this country. That is, it's a system for seeing the behaviors and reactions in your child and for categorizing their symptom profiles. They are categories, and they can't capture your child's humanity.

What is a mental disorder? You may be surprised to learn that no biological test can prove that a particular *mental disorder* exists, which is quite different from certain physical conditions, such as asthma or diabetes. But a system has developed for use in this country only. The American Psychiatric Association defines, lists, and classifies mental health disorders in the *Diagnostic and Statistical Manual of Statistical Disorders* (the *DSM* for short).[2] Such a system gives the medical doctors and psychiatrists who make up the American Psychiatric Association and other types of mental health professionals a common language of terms they can use to communicate.

I learned to do diagnosis and clinical assessment in my master of social work (MSW) program, and three years later, I was required to assign diagnoses during my family therapy postgraduate training program and have been using the *DSM* off and on ever since. The practical reason for diagnosis is that it is how mental health professionals, agencies, and facilities are paid through third-party payers, namely insurance companies and Medicaid.

Some parents feel relief when their child is diagnosed: finally, an explanation for why their child is acting in such baffling and frustrating ways. Other children share this particular emotional, mental, and behavioral profile. You can read and learn more about it, which may give a measure of control. The most important reason, of course, for a diagnosis is that it should inform treatment. But, along with good reasons for having the *DSM*, an established behavioral profile subject to research, and a means to provide for reimbursement of services, there are also some problems with this system.

Problems with the Concept of "Diagnosis"

After explaining this background and basis, I must offer some caution about the concept of "diagnosis," the *DSM* manual as its basis, and how medicine is practiced in this country.[3] First, the *DSM* is based on what's called a "categorical" system, meaning that symptoms that have persisted are counted up to determine whether criteria are met for that disorder category. For example, a major depressive disorder involves at least five symptoms lasting for two weeks. Categories tend to be a crude way to measure and assess. Sometimes people comment that categories put "people into boxes," which may be considered confining and restrictive. Therefore, diagnoses don't take into account the complexity of human beings. Children with the same diagnosis, for example, may look very different, making comparisons across children and how they respond an ongoing challenge.

A second problem with the *DSM* is that it promotes an arbitrary medical model of disorders as residing within clients. Many have criticized the tendency of psychiatry, coming as it does from the medical profession, to overstate the case for biological causation. Although the field of neuroscience, the study of the brain, has made advances, no definitive biological markers exist for any of the disorders.[4] Mental disorders are often described as chemical imbalances in the brain. That might be a useful way to think about them, but the brain and the complexity of neural functioning make it impossible to reduce disorders to a few neurochemicals that might be off kilter. Understand that a "disorder" doesn't exist as an objective reality—it's not something we can see and touch. Rather, it is a concept that may be more or less helpful to understand your child's and your experiences.

Beyond biology and the brain, it's probably more useful to think of mental disorder as arising from the reciprocal interactions between the child, including developmental, biological, and psychological influences, and the environment, including the immediate social system and wider social and cultural influences. In other words, mental disorder is a bio-psycho-social phenomenon rather than only a medical diagnosis. Because the medical profession formulates the way diagnoses are made, the interpersonal problems and stressful life events that may play a role aren't part of diagnosis and, therefore, are not reimbursable by insurance. In other words, the system of diagnosis enforces the medical view that a child's behavior is purely internal dysfunction.

Additionally, the *DSM* is a major moneymaker for the American Psychiatric Association. The revisions to the manual mean that every US mental health practitioner has to keep up to date by accessing or purchasing the manual, which, at this writing, costs $35. That doesn't count all the other supplementary materials associated with each new version, which include desk references, tabs, case study texts, handbooks, videos, and other types of training materials, including professional development seminars. In other words, each version spawns a lucrative publishing venture.

Perhaps most disturbing about the *DSM* is the way it furthers the purposes of pharmaceutical companies. As more constellations of behaviors are considered "mental disorders," there are more opportunities for treatment with medication. Drug companies benefit financially as more reimbursable disorders are made available. Drug companies sponsor research on medications, block unfavorable results from publication, fund psychiatric conferences and continuing education programs, and are major advertisers. The budget for marketing in pharmaceutical companies far outstrips their funding for research. They would rather sell what they already have or develop slight variations of what has been profitable for their competitors than finding new, possibly more effective treatments for people suffering with mental and emotional pain, among other common medical afflictions.[5]

As an example, the *New York Times* wrote a series in the early 2000s on the rapid rise of child bipolar diagnosis, a very serious mental illness.[6, 7, 8] One psychiatrist apparently was involved in aggressively disseminating pharmaceutical-funded research about the use of antipsychotic medication for youth believed to have bipolar disorder. He had not disclosed his association with the pharmaceutical company, although he was being handsomely compensated.

This particular situation is one that encouraged a change in policy. Now, in every article published, authors are required to disclose their connections to pharmaceutical companies. Such disclosures, however important, still don't change the symbiotic relationship that exists between doctors and pharmaceutical companies. As examples, pharmaceutical representatives visit psychiatrists' offices, take them out for meals, and provide other perks to woo business. Pharmaceutical companies also provide free continuing education and other bonuses to doctors who prescribe and feature their products.

Aside from this serious concern, the *DSM* promotes itself on the virtue of science, but many decisions about what to include and not include in the manual are made through changing social mores as much as anything else. For example, post-traumatic stress disorder was included because of the experience of military veterans, and homosexuality was taken out in 1974 with societal recognition that it wasn't a disorder.

Another surprising fact is the lack of a scientific basis to some disorders. An example is the newly created disruptive mood dysregulation disorder, an increasingly common disorder (see chapter 7). Overall, the reliability for many of the disorders is low, meaning that different providers give different diagnoses when presented with a case scenario without a great deal of agreement. This explains why the diagnoses for your child may shift by provider or over time.

Another reason for the different diagnoses your child may receive is for reimbursement purposes. A more severe diagnosis may be submitted by your child's psychiatrist because there is a need to justify for third-party payers the medication being prescribed. That same child may earn a much less severe disorder, such as an adjustment disorder, from an outpatient psychotherapist. Therefore, a diagnosis can be manipulated for the reimbursement of particular services.

We're taking the disorders one by one because that's how they're assigned, but your child might have an alphabet soup of labels. With that many, a level of imprecision is present, an anagram of trying to describe a child's observable symptoms. It's rare when there is only one diagnosis present in a child with a diagnosis.

A final problem with the *DSM* is that it says little about underlying reasons for symptoms. A diagnosis is based on clinical judgment about a certain symptom profile (e.g., "is my child forgetful," "is my child disorganized") without taking into account *why* your child is acting in a certain way. Most parents are concerned about the *why*s and what they can do about those, but a diagnosis may not reveal much about this key aspect.

SUMMARY

Although this book is organized by diagnosis because that's how you may access the mental health system and how providers speak, the diagnosis does not define your child. I find it more helpful to think about mental disorder in terms of a biological-psychological-social phenomenon. While your child may have certain vulnerabilities, there are also resources and strengths that you can access and bolster for your child at different system levels—in other words, there are environmental supports that can help your child function optimally. And you, as a parent or caregiver, are central to your child's environment. You are the most important person to your child even if it doesn't feel like it or your child actively tells you they hate you.

I want you to take away one core message from this information: A diagnosis is a useful shorthand to communicate with providers and others, and for getting services, but your child is much more than a simple checklist of symptoms. Indeed, you will see me use the word *the* in front of the diagnosis label at times. The reason for that is to discourage too much identity with the disorder. Your child is *not* the diagnosis; the word *the* externalizes the diagnostic label into its own entity rather than being seen as part of your child's core identity.

I am writing this book for parents—and other caregivers—of children with emotional and behavioral challenges who are having daily difficulties and are afraid of what the future will bring. This book will show you what help and supports are available and how to access them so your child and family life can be successful and rewarding. The mission of this book is to help you cope and to provide realistic information about the disorders, relying heavily on the research but also tempering with my personal and clinical experience.

PART I

Neurodevelopmental Disorders

Chapter 1

Attention-Deficit Hyperactivity Disorder

If your child has been diagnosed with attention-deficit hyperactivity disorder (ADHD), or you suspect ADHD, your child is certainly not alone. Six million youth ages four to seventeen, or 9 percent of youth in the United States, have been so diagnosed.[1] Rates have gone up over recent years (particularly since 2003). The reasons for the rising number of ADHD diagnoses may include:[2]

- Policy changes involving the Individuals with Disabilities Education Act
- Changing diagnostic criteria that make it easier for a child to meet the symptom threshold
- Changing social mores about childhood behavior
- The marketing efforts of pharmaceutical companies
- More youth entering college and, therefore, a greater need for students to do well academically

The prevalence of the disorder varies depending where in the world you live. In Europe, rates of diagnosis are lower than they are in the United States. European countries rely on the International Classification of Diseases (ICD) criteria, published by the World Health Organization, and use the nomenclature *hyperkinetic disorder*, which requires a more severe and extreme threshold of behavior. As a result, fewer children are diagnosed in those countries, although rates have increased there, as well. Even within the United States, the number of children diagnosed with ADHD varies widely by region[3]—rates are higher in southern and midwestern states than elsewhere in the country—and ethnicity—rates are lower for ethnic minority (Black and Latinx) children than white youth.[4] ADHD is more common in boys.

WHAT DOES ADHD LOOK LIKE?

Of course, all children—and adults—show hyperactive, impulsive, and inattentive behavior at times. Still, ADHD is characterized by the extreme and pervasive nature of these tendencies to the point where there is impairment in at least two settings, most typically home and school, for at least six months.[5]

There are three possible subtypes of ADHD:[6]

1. *Hyperactivity/impulsive type* with at least six of the following presenting "often": fidgeting; getting out of the seat when remaining seated is the expectation; runs about or climbs inappropriately; unable to play/engage in leisure activity quietly; talks excessively; blurts out; difficulty waiting for turn; interrupts; and is often "on the go."
2. *Inattentive type* with at least six of the following symptoms presenting "often": fails to give close attention to details or makes careless mistakes; difficulty sustaining attention to tasks; doesn't seem to listen when spoken to; doesn't follow through on instructions and tasks; difficulty organizing tasks and activities; avoids and dislikes tasks that require mental effort; loses things; easily distracted; forgetful.
3. *Combined type* in which the child meets criteria for both of the above.

In the *DSM* definition of mental disorder, impairment as a result of symptoms is required. Academic underperformance is typically present. Focus, concentration, self-control, and organization are all critical skills for academic success, and these are areas in which the child struggles. Children's behavior problems—inability to stay seated, blurting out, disrupting others' learning—also interfere with school performance. Problems with classmates and other peers are another possible area of impairment. Children who are impulsive, don't think before they act and speak, and have poor frustration tolerance and boundaries can be annoying to be around, even for other children. As I'm sure you know, family relationships are also often negatively impacted.

Aside from the symptoms themselves, there are other common problems. Approximately 20–50 percent of children diagnosed with ADHD have sleep problems, which may relate to the close connection in the brain between areas related to regulation of attention/affect and of sleep/arousal.[7] Additionally, a common side effect of stimulant medication is that it inhibits sleep.

Children with ADHD have a greater risk of breaking bones due to impulsivity. In the three years I saw a young girl in therapy for ADHD, she often showed up after having been to the ER for falls and sprains. Feelings of frustration and impatience can sometimes lead to outbursts and tantrums. The lack of emotional regulation may contribute to impulsive and reactive aggression.

Over time, some children develop self-esteem issues. They start to think of themselves as "stupid" because what seems to come easily to others is difficult for them. It's one of the frustrations of parenting such a child. With all the potential you see in your child, you wonder why they don't just try harder. But the inability to sustain effort is what is difficult in ADHD.

WHAT IT'S LIKE TO PARENT THIS CHILD

The study that formed the basis for this chapter involved my gathering and synthesizing interviews with parents who were raising children diagnosed with ADHD from studies published in the academic literature. I ended up finding eighty studies and analyzed the interviews for shared ideas.[8] One salient theme was the level of stress and anguish parents experienced, which seemed to be worse than for parents of children diagnosed with either autism or intellectual disorder.

Caregiving was experienced as a "24-hour a day" undertaking. As one mother of a seven-year-old said, "To be a teacher, mother, minder, carer, everything and twenty-four [hours] round the clock, it's just an exhausting experience." Another said, "a constant struggle always, always with her, every single day," while another said, "You feel like you are constantly on them all the time, nag-nag-nag. That can be sometimes a terrible feeling." Typical family routines, getting ready in the morning, doing homework in the afternoon, running errands, and bedtime routines, were an ongoing and daily challenge. As one mother reported, "It is very hard for my son to follow the daily routine, such as abiding by the daily rules and finishing his work at hand."

Many parents in my study talked about the difficulty of ordinary routines. One parent described: "Nothing is easy and I'm not only talking about schoolwork, I'm talking about if I need to run an errand after school. If I haven't prepped him for it in advance there can be a meltdown and lot of times, you can't do it. Or, if you do it, you pay the consequences of whiny, pain-in-the-ass crying. So I have to think very carefully about what needs to be done when they come home from school, so I can give them time to adjust to what we have to do. Sometimes that doesn't even work . . . I always have to be thinking. I always have to be planning . . . I have to do even more of that than most mothers. So it's difficult."

If you're a parent of a child with ADHD, you have to work harder than parents of children without the disorder to finesse situations to set your child and family up for success.[9] These daily negative interactions and behavioral management requirements demand considerable parental resources. The stress can be worse with male children and when hyperactivity is present. Many parents experience anxiety, depression,[10] frustration, exhaustion, isolation, grief, and even, in some cases, suicidality.[11] Guilt is often common. Some parents blame themselves for causing the ADHD, for failing to get help earlier, and for not being more patient.

The challenges of parenting spill into other areas, including a toll on health, job performance if you work outside the home, whether you can hold employment, and your relationship with your spouse or partner. Parents report that their children's relentless misbehavior negatively affects their marital and partner relationships. Children's need for constant attention often disrupts parents' time together. Second, mothers alone often play the role of disciplinarians. Fathers in studies sometimes lacked the effort and finesse required to manage these children effectively. A theme in some studies is that fathers perhaps have undiagnosed ADHD themselves and, therefore, were unable to provide the needed patience, organization, and structure.

You may recognize yourself in some of these reactions and realities, and rather than being depressing or demoralizing, I want this information to serve as validation for your struggles that other parents may not understand. You are not alone, and others are similarly struggling. Later in the chapter, I'll talk about some of the things that you can do to care for yourself amid this stress.

WHAT CAUSES ADHD?

The theory is that ADHD is primarily a problem of executive functioning[12] involving the more evolved parts of the brain related to regulating thoughts and behaviors. These include:

1. working memory: the capacity to hold information active in the mind and mentally work with it to guide behavior. For ADHD, this incapacity partly explains the forgetfulness that children with ADHD often show. They forget their backpacks, their clothes, their sports equipment, and their homework. I'm sure you've heard the phrase, often said in total exasperation, "He'd forget his head if it wasn't tied to him!" The working memory impairment is also why memorization, which is still required in schools, is difficult for your child, coupled with the lack of ability to sustain effort.
2. inhibition: the ability to override a habitual but incorrect response. This means that even when children have been taught and corrected, they have a difficult time learning. They still get caught up with their impulses and what is immediately in front of them.
3. mental set-shifting: the ability to flexibly switch between tasks or mental sets. This can explain some of the rigidity in approaching problems rather than being able to consider other options.

There is some evidence for this model of ADHD. Brain function (MRI technology) studies show that inattention and impulsivity deficits are associated with parts of the brain that involve impairments in cognitive function.[13] But MRIs aren't done routinely and are not used for diagnosis.

ADHD is believed to be inherited—40 percent of parents of children with ADHD may have a diagnosis of ADHD.[14] Therefore, if your child meets criteria, one parent or close relative (grandparents, cousins) may also fit the diagnosis, although likely remained undiagnosed because of a lack of recognition of the disorder at that time.

Despite the theory about ADHD being a heritable disorder, the science has not yet been able to identify the precise genes involved,[15] but what are called dopamine and serotonin transmitter and receptor genes have been linked to the disorder.[16] Neurotransmitters are chemical substances that pass messages from one neuron to another in the brain.

Aside from genetics, other biological pathways may influence the development of ADHD:

- premature birth[17]
- maternal smoking or drinking during pregnancy[18]
- prepregnancy obesity and overweight
- pre-eclampsia
- pregnancy complications
- paternal and maternal depression[19]
- maternal hormonal contraception use[20]
- maternal hypertension
- acetaminophen (e.g., Tylenol) exposure in the womb[21]
- lead exposure, which still can be present in low socioeconomic housing[22]
- environmental toxins, including what are called organophosphate pesticides, at levels common among US children.[23]

If you are pregnant or considering another pregnancy, these are conditions and exposures to avoid, if possible.

Parenting is *not* the cause of ADHD in children, although severe attachment situations, such as institutional care or late adoption, may give rise to symptoms in children, operating, it is believed, through neurological pathways and brain development. I saw a nine-year-old girl, Ioana, who spent the first year of her life in a Romanian prison where her mother gave birth. Ioana lay on her back for most of that time, to the point where her head was flattened, until she was transferred to an orphanage when her mother's parental rights were terminated. A couple in the United States adopted her at eighteen months, and she met full criteria for ADHD at a very young age.

HOW DO I GET THE DIAGNOSIS FOR MY CHILD?

The process of diagnosing children in the United States is not a standardized process and involves various providers and systems. Due to young children's short attention span and high energy levels, diagnosis often occurs when they start elementary school and encounter increased demands.

Primary Care Doctors

Pediatric doctors are primarily responsible for diagnosing ADHD in the United States. The advantage of this practice is that pediatricians presumably already know your child, and possible physical bases for symptoms have been eliminated. In any assessment for ADHD or other mental disorder, a physical exam and labs are necessary to rule out any conditions that might mimic or explain symptoms. Another advantage to a pediatrician diagnosis is that medication can be prescribed. If your child responds to the stimulant the doctor prescribes, then all is good. However, it can sometimes not be so easy to get a good response. At that point, pediatricians, rightly so, suggest a specialist in child psychiatry.

Because of efforts to improve the way primary care providers perform diagnoses, the Academy of Pediatrics has set up guidelines for pediatricians to follow. Most doctors now follow the *DSM* criteria and ask for teachers to complete rating scales so they get this critical input. Teachers, in fact, probably because of their experience with children, are more accurate than parents at identifying children's ADHD. However, due to time constraints—sessions are often scheduled at fifteen-minute increments—and lack of training, primary care providers are sometimes ill equipped to assess and manage a mental health disorder. Therefore, much variation exists among providers. As a result, ADHD is overdiagnosed—given to those who meet few symptoms—and underdiagnosed—not given to those who meet full criteria.[24] There are some interesting regional differences, with more children in the

South and Midwest diagnosed than in other parts of the country and more rural compared to urban children.

Psychiatrists

Psychiatrists are medical doctors who have an additional residence in psychiatric training. Currently, the vast majority of psychiatrists only prescribe medication and do not undertake any of the psychotherapy. There is a severe lack of child psychiatrists in the United States, particularly in certain states and rural areas. Because of the shortage, it may be difficult to find a psychiatrist who is taking new patients, depending on your area. In some major urban areas, like the DC metro area where I live, most psychiatrists do not accept insurance and ask for the full fee at the time of service, which may run in the hundreds for the initial consult and often around $250 for each fifteen- to thirty-minute follow-up session.

The benefits of psychiatrists are that they have received specialized training on mental disorders, and their practice centers around prescribing medication for these conditions. A psychiatrist generally may take a forty-five-minute session to diagnose ADHD. Hopefully, they will also get input from the teacher in the form of a questionnaire, as well as parent and child reports.

Because of the shortage of prescribers, other medical professionals, namely nurse practitioners and physicians' assistants with a psychiatric specialization, are supplementing the work of psychiatrists. Nurse practitioners have a doctoral degree, and physicians' assistants have a master's degree with an additional specialization in psychiatric practice.

Psychologists

Doctoral-level psychologists (PhD) have been specifically trained in psychological testing. In a psychoeducational assessment, a psychologist performs a whole battery of tests to assess your child's intellectual functioning, cognitive processing, working memory, and potential learning disorders. Depending on the school district and if your child's school performance has been affected (failing grades), the school might have a school-based psychologist perform the testing for your child. If the school doesn't do this, you have to get private testing done for your child. Some insurance plans pay partly for these, but they can cost a couple of thousand dollars out of pocket. If there is an ADHD diagnosis (or other diagnoses) in the report, the school has to abide by the documentation. Understand that while psychologists are experts in the assessment of ADHD and other related conditions, they cannot prescribe medication.

In my opinion, getting a psychoeducational assessment by a psychologist is the most thorough out of the possibilities I've covered here. It rules out other conditions and will pick up on other reasons for symptoms, such as a learning disability. It will also provide needed documentation for the school to determine the best services for your child.

Testing and School Services

The school may approve testing through their in-house psychologist if there is cause. Parents or other concerned adults can send a letter to the school requesting that a child be evaluated due to the impact on grades and ability to remain in the classroom. Legally, as a result of your documentation, the school has to hold an interdisciplinary meeting involving the principal or assistant principal; a school counselor; the social worker; a teacher; and the parents to determine whether there is "cause" to take this further.

HOW IS THE DIAGNOSIS OF ADHD MADE?

The diagnosis of ADHD is made based on observable behaviors and symptoms rather than any biological test, despite the presumed underlying neurological basis. Therefore, the diagnosis will not get at any underlying causes. In assessment, the provider will make what's called *differential diagnosis* between ADHD and other disorders, although children with ADHD are often also diagnosed with other disorders,[25] particularly oppositional defiant disorder (ODD) or conduct disorder (CD).[26] I cover ODD and CD in greater detail in chapters 7 and 8. For now, understand that the distinguishing feature between the two disorder types is that children with ODD/CD behave in a way that purposely provokes, annoys, and antagonizes others, whereas ADHD symptoms are not willful. As part of gathering information, the practitioner must explore the possibility of trauma history. Some of the symptoms of post-traumatic stress disorder (PTSD) may mimic those of hyperactivity: impulsivity, inattention, and inability to focus.[27] (See chapter 6.)

Girls

ADHD is more commonly diagnosed in boys, which might involve actual differences between genders, but girls also may be underdiagnosed.[28] Compared to boys, who tend toward higher energy levels, even girls with ADHD do not seem as active. Additionally, girls are more likely to have the inattentive type of ADHD. They may daydream and be distracted but are not disruptive and, therefore, are not as apt to garner the attention of school personnel. In fifth grade, Mabel went through a thorough psychoeducational assessment at the school, and the psychologist said it was inconclusive whether she had ADHD or not. Mabel's mother reported that her daughter was surprisingly *inactive* compared to other children. However, her forgetfulness, lack of organization, difficulties with short-term memory, distractedness, and daydreaming contributed to poor school performance over the subsequent years. At fourteen, she was diagnosed with ADHD by a psychiatrist. When she became old enough to self-report more accurately, she identified very much with the symptoms of ADHD and believed that it accounted for many of her challenges. Providers need to identify ADHD in girls when it exists. The Berkeley Girls with ADHD Longitudinal Study found that girls and women with ADHD had significant impairments into early adulthood if they were not treated.[29]

Ethnic Minorities

If you identify as Black or Latinx, it is key that your child is assessed carefully for the presence of ADHD symptoms as studies have indicated cultural biases in diagnosis.[30] Specifically, providers may overdiagnose disruptive behavior disorders, attributing behavioral challenges to criminality rather than ADHD.[31] There also may be cultural patterns to parenting beliefs, such as attributing ADHD symptoms to poor parenting or to a normal developmental stage that will be outgrown.[32] Recognize that ADHD is often a diagnosis that requires some parental advocacy to procure, either by advocating through the school, obtaining private testing, or the like.

Age of Child to Classmates

One factor that is a common source of *misdiagnosis* of ADHD involves the age of children relative to their classmates.[33] Their teachers identify children who are the youngest in their classes as having more ADHD symptoms.[34] The youngest kindergartners were 60 percent more likely to be diagnosed with ADHD than the oldest children in the same grade. Similarly, when that group of classmates reached the fifth and eighth grades, the youngest were more than twice as likely to be prescribed stimulants. This misdiagnosis likely accounts for about 20 percent—or 900,000—of the 4.5 million children currently identified as having ADHD.

There are a couple of implications from these research findings. First, you, as the parent, can be aware of this fact before trying to get your child diagnosed. Second, if you're reading this before your child has entered school, you may want to consider waiting for him or her, if on the younger side, to enter kindergarten until they're in the next grade level. Third, if your child is young for the age cutoff and showing a lot of hyperactive and inattentive symptoms in relation to peers, one option is to keep them back in the lower grade. There are often self-esteem consequences of such a move, so if you consider doing this, you will likely have to consider switching your child to another school entirely. It's a little trickier for girls since you don't know when puberty will hit. If a girl is held back to catch up to her peers in terms of attention, she may develop earlier than her peers, which is in itself a risk for some other disorders. This option has to be thought out carefully to make a risk-benefit decision.

COMING TO TERMS WITH THE DIAGNOSIS

Despite the popular lay opinion that ADHD is overdiagnosed and is an excuse for children acting out, parents with children who are diagnosed with ADHD do not accept the diagnosis lightly, and a lengthy processing period is often involved. For some parents, the label of ADHD will reduce self- and child-blame, as well as guilt. Their attributions for child behavior might shift. Before, their children seemed to have intention behind their behaviors: *They can control it if they want to.* But seeing the condition as neurological, parents might view behavior as outside the child's control. In my study, Darren, a parent of a nine-year-old, said, "He can't stop. He can't. I used to think that he didn't want to. That is, could he be deaf? Could he have a problem that he doesn't . . . ? But, the point is that he can't stop. He starts and it is tralalalala. Without being able to, he cannot control himself. That is what I now see."

Parents described an ongoing process of understanding and making sense of their children's ADHD diagnosis. As one mother put it, "Maybe that's his personality, maybe that's ADHD, maybe ADHD is personality and vice versa, I genuinely don't know."

As many parents do, you may struggle to find the parameters around the ADHD behavior and underlying causes and to what to attribute certain behaviors. Some parents have difficulty finding the line between what is normal for a particular developmental stage or for being a boy and abnormal behavior. This may be particularly difficult for dads. Some parents yearn for more definitive information, wondering, *what's really going on with my child?*

INTERVENTION

Receiving intervention in childhood appears to affect long-term functioning positively.[35] ADHD is considered a chronic condition, requiring ongoing management and monitoring. That is, treatment will not "cure" ADHD. What it can do is help your child cope with the challenges of focusing, organizing, and controlling energy; to compensate for the challenges; and prevent problems in the future.[36] Both psychosocial intervention and medication are options for treatment. Generally, almost two-thirds (62.0 percent) of youth take medication, and slightly less than half (46.7 percent) receive therapy.[37] In this chapter, school interventions are discussed initially because they are so salient for children. Medication is discussed next as the first-line intervention for ADHD, according to the research.

Working with the School

Under the Individuals with Disabilities Education Act (IDEA) of 1990 (the reauthorization of the Education for All Handicapped Children Act, PL 94–142), ADHD may qualify children for special education and accommodations under a classification called "other health impairment" when symptoms affect school performance. The IDEA further provides free and appropriate public education for children with ADHD.[38]

504 Accommodations

School-based accommodations for ADHD, called a "504," involve altering the delivery of academics, such as by adjusting the following while still retaining the content:[39]

- Scheduling: time and a half for tests
- Test setting: testing alone or in a small group setting
- Presentation style
- Response format

Unfortunately, many accommodations do not have a research basis, except for reading aloud test responses, and youth, parents, teachers, and administrators, when surveyed, indicate ambivalence and dissatisfaction with establishing accommodations. Accommodations should be implemented on a time-limited basis and assessed regularly to determine if they improve students' school performance.[40] Long-term use of blanket accommodations may create unintended dependence on them. Classrooms are often run with some kind of behavioral management system, and research supports this practice. Also helpful for child school performance is training children with ADHD in organizational skills and offering homework support.[41]

Individualized Education Plan

The school by law has to provide more services beyond a 504 if a child has an Individualized Education Plan (IEP). IEPs aren't typically granted for children who have ADHD unless they have other learning impairments. In a study comparing children with ADHD with an IEP to those who did not have one, there were no differences, even in learning disorders or behavioral profiles, except for lower academic performance among those with an IEP.[42] Generally, the school is more willing to become involved when the symptoms result in failing grades, although there are widespread differences in how individual schools enact the federal laws. This website gives parents much more information about how to obtain an IEP: https://www.understood.org/en/articles /evaluation-rights-what-you-need-to-know?fbclid=IwAR03Ixwt6Aqc -Vrp05YEDf0blWDdTGhUMWBgWSIUAEiNDHM8RuJrys2L8zM.

Suspensions

Many parents struggle when the school constantly calls them to pick their children up for various infractions. A way to curb this habitual reaction from the school is to request that a suspension letter be prepared for when you arrive. School officials understand that if there are letters documenting that your child cannot function in a mainstream classroom, they will have to provide more resources so that your child can receive an education. Your making this request will ensure that school personnel are not being reactive about a particular incident with your child and getting carried away in the moment with consequences and that, instead, this suspension is called for.

Type of School

Some parents consider taking their child out of public school and into a private one that is more "traditional" with smaller class sizes. However, private schools aren't always well equipped with resources to manage students of all different abilities and needs. The public school system, funded as it is by the government, has more resources and is held accountable to the legal standard. Generally speaking, a public school will be able to serve your child with ADHD better than a private one unless a private school is geared toward children with these kinds of disabilities. And, of course, private school is not often free, so the cost may be prohibitive and may not provide the best services.

Medication

Medication is the most effective treatment option for addressing core symptoms of ADHD[43] and is considered a first-line intervention. Note that most of the gold standard research involves a few-week period in which stimulants are tested against a pill placebo. In contrast, children often take medication for an extended time frame, perhaps years, due to the chronic nature of the disorder.[44] In an excellent resource about ADHD medications, *ADHD Medication: Does it Work?*, Dr. Walt Karniski presents evidence of brain structural changes from consistent medication use that may account for the positive changes in focus and attention.[45] In other words, based on his clinical wisdom and the research, he is adamant that long-term use has benefits.

The psychostimulants are the largest class of medications prescribed for ADHD. These include methylphenidate (e.g., Ritalin), which has been used for decades, and the more recently popular amphetamines (e.g., Adderall).[46] Understand that all the stimulants are based on these two compounds, although delivery methods may differ (pill, liquid, patch), and various formulations may now be extended-release (seven to ten hours). There are currently over forty different medications for ADHD. However, the recommendation is to start with methylphenidate because it has been around the longest, has been most thoroughly researched, and may induce a smoother transition once the medication wears off than the amphetamines.[47] The Children and Adults with Attention-Deficit/Hyperactivity Disorder (CHADD) organization has an excellent chart that lists all the variations of methlyphenidate and amphetamines that your doctor may describe: https://chadd.org/wp-content/uploads/2021/09/ADHD-MEDICATIONS-APPROVED-BY-THE-US-FDA-2021.pdf. This chart displays the brand and chemical names, dosage, and form they take (capsule, pill, liquid). Nowadays, there are both regular or short-acting formulations, which may have to be taken more than once a day (such as at lunchtime at school or in the afternoon after school), or extended-release formulations that last for most of the day.

Some children don't respond to the stimulants, or the side effects are too difficult to live with. Common stimulant alternatives include atomoxetine (Strattera), a selective norepinephrine reuptake inhibitor (SNRI), and guanfacine (Tenex or Intuniv) and clonidine (Catapres or Kapvay), both originally designed to lower blood pressure. Guanfacine and clonidine are believed to work on the part of the brain related to impulsivity and attention. They are taken at nighttime and are sometimes used for sleep problems.

Doctors prescribe medication based on their clinical experience with many patients. Pharmaceutical representatives may also influence them to offer one drug over another. The type they prescribe may also be based on your child's needs. For instance, if your child has difficulty swallowing pills, they may offer a liquid alternative, such as Quivallent. Sometimes, a medication is chosen because you have a relative that has responded well to one in particular, as there's an assumption of shared genetics.

Stimulants are classified as Schedule II drugs by the Drug Enforcement Agency, along with cocaine and methamphetamine, because of their abuse potential. Schedule II is the most restrictive classification for medications, prohibiting both their prescription by phone and the writing of refills. As with all psychotropic medicines, those used for treating mental disorders, it is often a trial-and-error process to see which medication and at what dose works best for your child. One development in the field has been gene testing to determine the drugs to which your child is likely to respond. That may reduce some guesswork involved with getting an effective medication to work. Ask your doctor if he/she can request this from your insurance company. More information is available on this type of testing here: https://www.mayo.edu/research/centers-programs/center-individualized-medicine/patient-care/pharmacogenomics.

Another consideration about medication has to do with the way it is provided. In the Multi-Modal ADHD Treatment Study (MTA), the largest controlled study on treatment for ADHD, medication was only superior to other treatments when dosages were monitored frequently and titrated upward to an optimal dose.[48] In regular community practice, titration of dosage occurs less than at recommended levels, suggesting that at least some children are not receiving optimal treatment.[49] This means you should have regular appointments, such as monthly at the beginning of treatment, to determine the optimal dosage. After your child has stabilized on a particular medication, you can go once every three months.

How Old Should Kids Be to Take Medicine?

For preschoolers, the American Academy of Pediatrics recommends a twelve-week course of parent-child interaction therapy, a type of parent management training focusing on behavioral techniques and the attachment relationship between parent and child (see chapter 2), as a first-line intervention. If behavioral interventions don't work to curb behaviors, methylphenidate (Ritalin) is the first choice,[50] as it has been the only drug studied with this age-group.[51] Many doctors will not prescribe until children are five and only in extreme cases.

Side Effects

Insomnia: As mentioned, sleep problems are already common for children with ADHD, and stimulant medication sometimes exacerbates this concern.[52] Sleep hygiene is an important first-line approach. Some of the elements involved are:

1. Perform a regular sleep routine, getting up and going to bed at roughly the same time each day, rather than having drastically different schedules on the weekdays compared to the weekends.
2. Have a relaxing routine in the evening—reading, bathing, crafts—so children start to wind down.
3. Don't allow children to hang out in their bed watching TV or being on a computer/tablet during the day. Otherwise, they will associate their beds with *not* sleeping.
4. Shut down electronic devices an hour before bedtime.
5. Don't have a TV or other media beyond audiobooks in children's rooms at night.
6. Have children get sufficient physical activity during the day.

These interventions should all be done before turning to supplements and medication, which many kids with ADHD take. As a parent said in my study, "Nighttime is bad because my son doesn't have a high sleep requirement. If he doesn't have his nighttime meds, he doesn't go to bed until midnight, one, two, three, four o'clock in the morning. He doesn't sleep without nighttime meds. Bedtime is the hardest because it's hard for them to calm down."

Many children with ADHD take the supplement melatonin for sleep. Melatonin mimics the hormone found in the brain that controls sleep-wake cycles. Although the warning on such supplementssays that they are only to be taken for a short time, children often take these nightly for potentially years, although this practice has yet to be researched. Other medications that doctors prescribe for sleep when children haven't responded to all of the above are the previously mentioned guanfacine or clonidine. Trazadone, initially formulated for depression, is now more commonly used for sleep difficulties than depression.

Related to problems sleeping are issues with getting up in the morning. Morning routines can be very difficult for parents with children diagnosed with ADHD.[53] As much as possible, take care of tasks the night before—gathering items together for the backpack, setting out clothes, making lunches—so that morning is not such a scramble. For younger children, having routines—getting dressed, eating breakfast, brushing teeth—can be spelled out in pictures that are placed in a visible spot that you can point to. Barkley, an authority on ADHD, suggests that children have their ADHD medication on the nightstand beside their bed. The first alarm is set for thirty minutes before they have to wake up, so they take their medicine then. When the second alarm goes off thirty minutes later, the medication should have kicked in, and they can get up more easily.

Appetite Suppression: Stimulants have the common side effect of suppressing appetite. In the past, variations of stimulants were used as diet aids. Parents have come up with a variety of ways to deal with this side effect, such as making sure their child eats a decent breakfast before the appetite-suppressing effects kick in, using short-acting formulations that wear off for dinner, and providing high-calorie drinks like Ensure and protein bars for kids to eat at lunch when the appetite-suppressing effect might be most potent. Methylphenidate has a less negative impact on appetite than do amphetamines.[54]

In a sixteen-year follow-up of the MTA study, the height and weight of adults medicated as children were examined.[55] Children who were consistently on medication over that period were both shorter at an average of one and a half inches and weighed more with greater body mass compared to those who had received negligible amounts of medicine or people who were selected from the community as comparisons. It's difficult to decide whether to medicate your children, and you need accurate information to make that choice given the risks and benefits. However, parents who had undiagnosed ADHD themselves as children often state that they wished they had been medicated so they could have fulfilled more of their potential and not have struggled to the degree they did for years.

Decision-Making About Medication

Despite the widespread perception that stimulant medication is over-used, parents in my study did not take lightly the decision to medicate their children. A typical initial experience was one of cautious reservation. One parent reported, "I know how difficult it is to decide about medication. I waited six months before I allowed my child to try the medication. I didn't want to try the medication before exhausting other options." Another parent with a similar sentiment said, "As she got older it was more apparent that I did really need to treat her symptoms to make her function in the classroom better, to feel better about herself, and more functional in our home and even outside our home, socially with peers or anyone, it had to happen."

Other parents only try medication as "a last resort." One parent explained, "We wished that we had been able to somehow find a way to manage this without medication, but clearly, that's not the case. We've done our best, given it our best shot, but our son is still suffering. We are gonna give it a trial of medication."

Some parents report relief after the child began taking medication. One parent explained, "I wouldn't be without it because he is so difficult without it." Most participants found benefits to medication, particularly the positive effects on school performance. But parents also complain about side effects, causing them to discontinue medication use entirely in some cases. The decision to start medication for ADHD is a trade-off between benefits and side effects.[56]

Psychosocial Intervention

Generally, *behavioral management training*, also called *parent training* and *contingency management*, is more effective than individual interventions with children. Children with ADHD don't tend to report their symptoms accurately, and their insight is low. Neither are they motivated to put effort toward changing and learning new behaviors. The fact that therapeutic efforts are directed at teaching discipline techniques that are effective with these kinds of behavioral challenges doesn't mean to imply blame, although it may not seem "fair" when your child is the one acting out, and you're already doing so much work.

Because this chapter has overlapping material with chapter 7 in terms of research-supported treatment for behavior problems, discipline strategies are detailed there. Behavioral parent training approaches are considered a well-established treatment[57] that is effective for ADHD in youth,[58] according to both parent and observational reports, and gains are maintained over follow-up intervals. In the United States, parent management training is the treatment of choice for young children, aged six to eight, and suggested for school-age and adolescent youth.[59] Younger children benefit more from parent training than do older youth.[60]

Being a researcher, I was impressed with the large body of research that supports behavioral management training, and in my experience with parents who implemented the techniques consistently, their child's behavior was better than it could have been. However, it didn't get their child to the "normal" functioning level and fell far short of what was desirable. Similarly, parents in my study corroborated that discipline techniques only worked in a limited capacity.[61] As one parent said, "There is no easy way to discipline an ADHD child." Another said, "It's very frustrating to figure out how to discipline this kid." Yet another reported, "We've tried a lot of different behavior programs." Parents spoke candidly about the level of structure necessary in their parenting approach. For some, this took so much work that family life felt mechanistic and sapped their enjoyment.

What Parents Can Do

Self-Care: Parenting in general takes a lot out of people in terms of effort, time, and resources. Parenting a child diagnosed with ADHD is on a whole other level. For the bid on your own resources, it's important to get breaks, support, and self-care.

Self-care, at its most basic level, is taking care of your health. It's important amid scheduling for your child that you don't neglect your own routine appointments, including wellness visits/gynecological exams, mammograms, dentist appointments, and so forth.

Part of taking care of your health is attending to any mental health challenges of your own, whether these preceded the ADHD diagnosis or arose in part because of parenting a child with a lot of demands. Therapy or medication might be indicated if you are struggling. You can't be a good support and ally for your child if you don't feel well yourself. Chapters 9 and 10 delve into the details of looking for qualified therapists, as well as how to pay.

I recognize time and resource constraints, at least in part due to the demands of the ADHD, but it's critical to add some regular "self-care" or replenishment, such as exercising, going to a gym, a daily mindfulness activity, spirituality/prayer, craft-making, movie-watching, gardening, a sport, massages, nights out with your partner or friends, or classes.

Coping: Craig and colleagues (2020), researchers from Italy, examined the coping resources of parents with children diagnosed with ADHD.[62] They found that parents could not always identify the ways they could cope and relied heavily on avoidance, which generally means denial, minimizing, or escaping the problem. The research differentiates *distraction*, which is a healthy way of coping, versus avoidance, which is not. *Distraction* is a temporary means of taking your mind off troubles that doesn't have any negative effects. For example, if playing video games is your thing, then playing a game for a while might help you feel a sense of enjoyment, and then you can come back to challenges feeling a bit more refreshed. Using the same example but for avoidance would be playing video games for hours on end, and not tending to responsibilities as a result. Your partner might be mad at you for not doing your share, and you might stay up too late and be unable to wake up on time to tend to obligations.

Physical Activity: You may have already done this out of necessity, but enroll your child early in sports and model and encourage physical activity outdoors, if possible. When Danielle's son was young, she signed him up for two sports each season. It helped him get some energy out, and he could socialize with other boys at the same time, which he enjoyed. Danielle could take a break from caregiving and chat with other parents. Even if common sense doesn't say that this is helpful, the research bears it out and has even identified a minimum— twenty minutes a day on any kind of exercise. Talia and her husband forced their twins who both had ADHD to do hikes on the weekends to tire out their energy. If you can gain this kind of cooperation and make it a routine, doing physical activity as a family is ideal.

Support—from your partner, family members, friends, colleagues, or something more formal—is essential. Many parents with kids diagnosed with disabilities don't find it helps much to talk to other parents who didn't have a frame of reference for mental health challenges. Trying to be helpful, some people minimize your difficulties, making statements such as, "All kids act like that." Again, the symptoms of ADHD do include the inattentive, impulsive, and hyperactive types of behaviors that almost all children show. It's the severity, pervasiveness, and extreme nature of this pattern that makes up the criteria for ADHD. You need a place where you can vent without judgment. If people say or imply that you are not disciplining properly or "loving them enough," these people may not be helpful recipients of your frustrations. Another option here is to set up any such conversation so that you ask for what you need in advance: "I'm struggling a bit and don't need advice, just a supportive ear."

At the end of this chapter, there are a list of potential support groups that you might find helpful, both online forums and more typical support groups. There are also formal supports you can access, such as therapy or a support group. Chapter 10 dives more deeply into parental assistance.

Partner Support: Research supports that parents who have a child diagnosed with ADHD are more likely to be divorced than parents without a child diagnosed. This pattern could be due to the stress on parents of having a child with these behaviors and the fact that parents often have different parenting styles. There is often a gender pattern in that moms are more lenient. They tend to be more supportive and empathic. If dads recognize they might have been diagnosed if they were born in a different time cohort, they can be empathic. But often dads may not "believe in ADHD," and instead think that stricter discipline will cure the child. Unfortunately, this isn't an uncommon pattern between parents. One plays "strict," and the other "lax," and then they argue over that, creating even more tension in the household. Children are clever about playing their parents down the middle. They will go to the more easygoing parent for requests, which are then difficult to take back.

What can you do? Certainly, communicate with your spouse or partner. Try to stick to "I" messages: "I feel worried that he learns that he can get what he wants by asking you even when I've said no. I feel frustrated that I have told him he has to wait to get this reward when his behavior is better, and I have to withstand his badgering. I feel sad that he looks at me like the 'bad guy,' and you get to be the 'good guy.'" It's important to be on the same team, however you can get there. Understandably, you may not want more appointments to set up and attend, but couples counseling may be a helpful option. See chapter 10.

Understand that your child's therapist can't undertake partner relationship work, and instead, you'll have to find a different therapist for that. Parenting a child may put stress on your relationship, and you have to be each other's support for the challenges you face.

Simplify the routine, so there are only basic demands on your child and, by extension, you. When Carlotta's son was a baby, he cried continuously in the car and the stroller, so she and her husband had their groceries delivered because even going to the store was too stressful. Even what we take for granted as simple errands can be difficult with an uncooperative child. Andrea tried to take her son with her to the post office. There was a long line, and he misbehaved as they waited to the point where one of the postal workers reprimanded him. When Andrea finally reached the window, he ran out of the post office. Too angry at that point, she finished up her business before going after him. When she went outside, she found that he'd climbed on top of their minivan. At that point, she realized that not only was it incredibly stressful trying to get tasks done with him, but it might even pose a safety risk.

When she went into stores with her mother, nine-year-old Sasha would demand things constantly—treats, balloons, stuffed animals—and make scenes, embarrassing her mom, who sometimes would give in to buying her stuff. Of course, this reinforced Sasha's tantrums. (More on this in chapter 7.) If behavior is this unmanageable, there may be a period of time when your child just has to stay home, and you go without them to get errands done.

Similarly, supposedly fun family activities and vacations are sometimes not fun with children with ADHD. Without meaning to, they might end up ruining the rest of the family's time. Despite how much children diagnosed with ADHD resist routines, they do better with regular structure. Being in a different place with different arrangements and schedules might overwhelm certain children so much that they become dysregulated and unmanageable.

Instead, consider "staycations" or undertake activities with a lot of support people in place. Some parents find that having the child's grandparents or other relatives involved on vacations helps steady the child and provides that extra support that is often needed. However, that will depend on how supportive relatives are.

Of course, none of this sounds enjoyable—paying a babysitter so you can get errands done, staying home rather than going places—but you have to weigh the potential gains with the drawbacks—tantrums, embarrassment, dysregulation of your child which might take hours to de-escalate, the damage to your own sense of well-being.

Your Employment: I found in my study that parents often had to cut back on hours or quit/change jobs to better manage their child's behavior, to be available to go to the school for meetings and pick up their children, and to schedule and ferry around their child to myriad medical appointments.

If you're having difficulty managing your employment situation, some things might help. First, as mentioned, ensure that you require the school to supply written documentation of a suspension. This request may ensure that they only suspend your child when necessary and/ or build a case that they need to do more for your child. Second, if you have missed significant work and could benefit from time off, an option is to apply for family leave from your employer. The Family and Medical Leave Act is federal legislation that involves unpaid leave taken for up to twelve weeks for a serious medical illness in an employee or a family member. The website https://www.dol.gov/agencies/whd/fmla gives more information about the policy and if it applies to you. A third option is to apply for Social Security Insurance, explained in chapter 9.

CONSIDERATIONS FOR TEENS

Before, the common belief was that teenagers outgrew ADHD, but about half to 80 percent of elementary school children are still diagnosed as adolescents. Teens with ADHD may show more risky behavior. Teenagers who drive are more likely to speed and get into car accidents, and teens with ADHD are more at risk for substance use problems. This may be because they use substances to calm themselves down or focus or because they are impulsive and lack the ability to self-control. They may also have co-occurring disorders, such as oppositional defiant disorder or conduct disorder, which means they enjoy risk-taking. Interestingly, teens who receive medication for ADHD are less likely to develop substance use disorders[63] than those who are untreated. But fewer than half (45 percent) of twelve- to seventeen-year-olds with ADHD report receiving medication during the past week.[64] Youth with

ADHD who receive medication are also less likely to show suicidality than their non-medicated counterparts.[65]

Pregnancy risk is high in adolescents with ADHD because of impulsivity. Therefore, parental monitoring, sex education, and contraceptive care are key.

In my opinion, it's not a good idea to share your impetuous youth with your children. I know why parents are tempted to do so. It's being honest, right? You don't want to come off as holier than thou. You want to be real for your kids. You also want to teach them that you have regrets about your behavior, and you're hoping to forestall your child from going through the same thing—a lesson in advance, if you will.

The problem with sharing details of your younger life involving sex, drugs, and alcohol is that it's a bit of a boundary problem; your child isn't your confidante, and they really don't want to know or see you in this light. Children also often later use those confessions to rationalize their behavior. It doesn't end up being the intended lesson; instead, children employ it as an excuse.

SUMMARY

This chapter has provided psychoeducation about ADHD, the importance of having this information, and how to best work with it to get a diagnosis if necessary and receive optimal services. Parenting stress is considerable with child ADHD, and validation, respite, and support are essential. Recognize that in most cases, ADHD in children will be accompanied by other disorders, so some of the behaviors you see may not be the ADHD itself. The information in other chapters will be relevant in these cases.

Chapter 2

Autism Spectrum Disorders

Individuals on the autism spectrum have a unique way of perceiving and engaging with the world, accompanied by distinct strengths and challenges that may necessitate support and accommodations. Autism spectrum disorder (ASD) is a neurological-developmental condition that emerges within the first three years of life. Two primary areas of development differ among individuals with autism.[1]

The first area involves social communication, encompassing difficulties with verbal expression, understanding others' emotions and nonverbal cues, and engaging in reciprocal conversations. Many children with autism face challenges deciphering other people's emotions and initiating, maintaining, and responding to communication attempts. Moreover, they may struggle with staying on topic and understanding others' perspectives. Interpreting nonverbal gestures like hand signals, nods, and facial expressions can pose challenges, and autistic individuals may exhibit either excessive or insufficient eye contact during social interactions. Ryan, a ten-year-old boy with autism, excitedly showed his uncle the crabs he had discovered at the beach. In response, his uncle exclaimed, "Get out of here!" Misinterpreting this expression, Ryan ran away down the beach. His father, who witnessed the incident, chased after him, while his uncle remained perplexed. This example underscores the significance of employing clear and literal language, as individuals with autism may struggle with figurative language and sarcasm.

The second area of divergence lies in restricted interests and repetitive behaviors, which may manifest as self-stimulatory actions or difficulties with transitions and unexpected schedule changes. Children with autism may interact with toys in unconventional ways, such as sorting them by size or color, arranging them in lines, or focusing on peculiar attributes. Additionally, they may exhibit an atypical fascination with objects that are typically uninteresting to other children, such as dishwashers, pencils, or state flags.

Children on the spectrum often find comfort in adhering to schedules, as they provide structure and predictability. Uncertainty may be challenging, while routines offer control over the environment, alleviate anxiety, and enable better preparation for forthcoming events or transitions. Seven-year-old Lauren strictly followed a precise bedtime ritual that she had to execute in a specific order: brushing with a red toothbrush, wearing a blue T-shirt, and reading a particular book before bed each night.

At the time of this writing, a newly proposed definition of autism, *profound autism*, describes a more severe form characterized by significant impairments in communication, social interaction, and behavior. Individuals with profound autism typically have little or no speech, limited social interactions, and repetitive behaviors.[2] They may also have intellectual disabilities (IQ <50), sensory sensitivities, and difficulty with changes in routine or environment. People with profound autism require extensive support and care throughout their lives. We suggest viewing *In A Different Key: The Story of Autism*, a PBS film that explores the history and impact of autism on individuals and society.[3] In the autism community, functioning labels are discouraged because they can be misleading, but this chapter includes supports that can be used at varying degrees for those with support needs, such as visuals, assisted communication, and social narratives.

DISABILITY LANGUAGE

Using person-first language, as in "child with autism," promotes respect and dignity for the individual and acknowledges an individual's worth beyond their diagnosis.[4] Many prefer disability identity-first language because it honors one's unique identity as an autistic person. When sixth-grade Sarah heard about person-first vs. identity-first language, she said, "No one has ever asked me that. I prefer to be called 'autistic.' Calling me a person with autism sounds weird and makes it seem like the autism is separate from who I am." Both disability-first and identity-first language have their proponents and critics, with ongoing debates about the more appropriate or respectful approach. Language preferences vary among individuals and should be respected to promote inclusivity. In this chapter, you'll notice that we use person- *and* identity-first language.

PREVALENCE

The prevalence of ASD is difficult to gauge due to differences in assessment techniques both worldwide and in the United States.[5] There is even diagnostic variability across states, which may relate to the training of professionals, the availability of pediatricians, and the accessibility of health care resources. According to the Centers for Disease Control, in 2023, the current autism prevalence rate is one in every thirty-six children, which equates to almost 3 percent of eight-year-olds.[6, 7] The estimated percentage has continued to increase over previous years' estimates. Among eight-year-old children, boys were nearly four times as likely as girls to be identified with ASD.

ASSESSMENT AND DIAGNOSIS

A significant thrust in health care is the early diagnosis of ASD so that intervention can begin as soon as possible.[8] The severity of symptoms and parental concern are essential factors in early identification. Ninety percent of parents recognize a difference in their child by twenty-four months.[9] During the first year of life, the child typically displays unusual social development, being less likely to imitate the movements and vocal sounds of others, and exhibits problems with attention and responding to external stimulation.[10] Between one and three years of age, when parents are most likely to seek evaluation, differences from peers are readily apparent, and the child's idiosyncratic, self-focused behaviors and communication differences can be striking. During an autism assessment when Kelly was six, her father remembered that she was a late talker, and he mentioned that he didn't think much of her unusually intense interest in state flags. He described her differences as noticeable during playgroups and social interactions but didn't pay much attention to these differences.

Neurologists and developmental pediatricians are often responsible for diagnosing ASD, with primary pediatricians doing so only 12 percent of the time.[11] Many children with ASD are initially evaluated at a mean age of forty-eight months but are not diagnosed until sixty-one months.[12] Most practitioners do not use a diagnostic screening instrument, and 20 percent to 25 percent of children are not diagnosed until after school entry.

Assessment is challenging because no biochemical tests are available, nor does a single behavior or set of behaviors characterize ASD. Assessment should be multidisciplinary, including evaluations by a clinical or school psychologist, medical doctor, speech and language pathologist, and a social worker. The assessment goals are to determine if a child has autism and then educate parents and caregivers that autism is a naturally occurring variation in human neurology that deserves acceptance and accommodations. Parents should seek professionals who use neurodiversity-affirming strategies, acknowledge child strengths and abilities, and highlight the unique qualities that make them who they are. Parents can learn from the neurodiversity movement and the diversity of experiences and perspectives within the autism community to help them understand autism as part of their child's identity and to support and celebrate neurodiversity.

A core assessment for ASD comprises the following elements:[13]

- Information from parents. Mom's pregnancy, labor, and delivery; the child's early neonatal course; the parents' earliest concerns about their child; family history of developmental disorders; symptoms in the areas of social interaction, communication/ play, and restricted or unusual interests; the presence of problem behaviors that may interfere with intervention, such as aggression, self-injury, and other behavioral oddities; and the child's prior response to any educational programs or behavioral interventions
- Direct observations in structured (school) and unstructured (home) settings and in interactions with peers, parents, and siblings
- Medical evaluation for possible seizures, visual and hearing examinations for possible sensory differences, and testing for lead levels if the child has had exposure
- Cognitive assessment for the level of intellectual functioning
- Assessment of adaptive functioning and social skill development

• Speech and language assessment.

WHAT CAUSES AUTISM?

Neurodiversity is a concept that recognizes and celebrates the natural variation in brain function and neurodevelopment among individuals. It emphasizes that neurological differences, such as autism, ADHD, dyslexia, and other conditions, are normal variations of human neurology rather than disorders or deficiencies. The neurodiversity movement promotes acceptance and inclusion of all neurologically diverse individuals in society, aiming to create an environment that values their diverse ways of thinking and processing information. It emphasizes the importance of accommodating and supporting the needs and strengths of neurodivergent individuals rather than trying to "normalize" or change them. That being said, we now cover some of the theories and science behind the development of autism specifically.

Biological

ASD is considered a neurodevelopmental disorder because of its high rates of heredity transmission.[14] For instance, 10 percent of siblings also develop ASD.[15] Many genes, perhaps as many as one hundred, contribute to the development of ASD.[16] Chromosomal damage appears to occur in genes that control growth and development in early life; influence speech and language development; cause behavioral symptoms associated with ASD; contribute to tuberous sclerosis (a disorder characterized by seizures and intellectual disability); are related to metabolic and serotonin deficiencies; and prompt the development of fragile X, a type of intellectual disability.

Advanced parental age (over age forty) in either mothers or fathers creates an increased risk.[17] Possible biological mechanisms here include chromosomal mutations associated with advancing age or alterations in genetic imprinting. Birth complications may contribute to risk, and other pregnancy-related factors—maternal obesity, maternal diabetes, and caesarean section—have shown a less intense but still significant association with the risk of ASD.[18] Environmental toxicants, at least for a subset of children, may have an equal contribution to the development of ASD as genetics.[19] Although some parents believe that vaccines are the cause of ASD, there is no scientific evidence to support the link.[20]

Protective influences, meaning factors that often lead to better outcomes in the long run, for the course of ASD include an absence of pregnancy and birth complications, a later age of onset (after twenty-four months), the child's early acquisition of nonverbal communication, functional play skills, speech capacity, milder level of impairment, and the absence of intellectual disability.[21, 22]

Social Influences

Social factors are involved, not in the development of autism itself, but when the diagnosis is made. Therefore, rest assured that no parenting factors have anything to do with the development of autism. Children from lower-income families may have a later diagnosis of autism.[23] Higher-income parents may be better able to navigate the medical system and have more access to resources that enable diagnosis.

Promote, if possible, the resilience factors for caregivers that are linked to better adjustment: the availability of social support, spousal support, having a sense of efficacy and optimism; and using reframing and acceptance.[24] Parents developed resilience as the child got older, and more time passed since the diagnosis.

A protective family factor that leads to better outcomes for the child involves high-quality parent-child interactions. When Rachel was diagnosed with autism at two, her mother, Sarah, felt overwhelmed, as if she needed to meet with every available therapist and doctor. Over time, Sarah connected with a therapist who offered parent training, which taught her helpful strategies that empowered her to be an active partner in her daughter's care.

INTERVENTIONS

Comprehensive interventions for children with ASD include strategies that address its core areas of communication, social interaction, and flexibility in thinking and behavior. The range of interventions can include behavior management, special education, family support, and support with social skills. As a parent, it's difficult to wade through all the available information and determine what is valid. A reliable online free source of support that explains strategies that are effective in helping children with autism is the Autism Focused Intervention Resources & Modules (AFIRM) at https://afirm.fpg.unc.edu,[25] and resources for evidence-based practices identified by the National Clearinghouse on Autism Evidence & Practice on Autism Spectrum Disorder are available at https://autismpdc.fpg.unc.edu/.

Ideas and therapies found online are not always researched; some may cause harm. For example, chelation therapy, gluten-free/casein-free diets, and hyperbaric oxygen therapy have no scientific evidence as effective treatments for autism.[26] Chelation therapy involves administering a chemical that can remove heavy metals from the body and can result in severe side effects such as organ damage, heart failure, and even death. Cutting out essential nutrients from your child's diet can lead to malnutrition and further developmental problems. Hyperbaric oxygen therapy involves being placed in a pressurized chamber and exposed to pure oxygen. It can result in side effects such as seizures, ear and sinus injuries, and oxygen toxicity.

Applied Behavior Analysis

Behavioral interventions focus on improving functioning and adaptation capacities. Applied behavior analysis (ABA) is a scientific and evidence-based approach to understanding how human behavior works. It focuses on identifying ways to improve positive behaviors and reduce negative ones through systematic observation, measurement, and analysis.[27] An ABA specialist works directly with the child and uses reinforcement, prompting, and shaping principles to teach individuals socially significant behaviors, such as communication, self-care, socialization, and academic skills. Reinforcement, a key principle in behavior therapy, is used to increase or strengthen behavior. Essentially, reinforcement means that whenever a child exhibits a desired behavior, they receive a positive consequence. For example, if your child puts away their backpack, you provide specific praise, "Great job putting your backpack away."

Prompting involves providing cues or hints to help your child understand expectations.[28] Prompts include moving an item closer to your child, using pictures or visuals, showing your child how to do something by modeling and pointing to something, or using language or reminders. For example, a therapist might tell your child, "Please pick up your cup." If, after a determined number of seconds, your child does not respond, the therapist will use a more supportive prompt and move the cup closer to your child. It's often used with positive reinforcement to encourage your child to engage in the desired behavior. Over time, as your child becomes more confident with their skills, prompts should gradually fade out, allowing your child to become more independent and self-sufficient.

While ABA has helped many children with ASD improve their behavior, critics say that the highly structured and regimented therapy sessions emphasize compliance and conformance rather than accommodating individual needs and preferences. They argue that it shouldn't be the only therapy option available, and must be approached with care and sensitivity to each child's needs.[29] Shirley, the mother of a three-year-old nonspeaking boy with autism, investigated behavioral treatment options and found an ABA therapist to work with her son in their home. She felt this was an ideal option for the family, as she felt more connected to the therapy process, and therapy goals felt natural as they related to home behaviors.

Parent Coaching or Mediated Interventions

Many therapies are parent mediated, meaning the parent or caregiver takes on a primary intervention role with the child and is trained in behavior techniques. These types of treatments enhance consistency in intervention at home and school and facilitate the child's generalization of skills across settings. Although they can't change the child's core symptoms, parent-mediated interventions (PMII) can enhance the child-parent relationship.[30] PMII makes parents active participants by teaching them behaviors or skills they can use during everyday activities and routines. The National Professional Development Center on Autism Spectrum Disorder report *Evidence-Based Practices for Children, Youth, and Young Adults with Autism* lists and describes various evidence-based models. If you find a model that might be helpful (e.g., Research Units in Behavioral Intervention [RUBI], Project ImPACT [PI], Triple P [Positive Parenting Program]), visit the particular model's webpage to search for a certified provider in your area.

Parent Support

Parents and caregivers can benefit greatly from educational and supportive interventions, particularly those in groups. Many parents share that they found it helpful to connect with other parents, even forging new friendships for themselves and their children. Many states have autism organizations that provide parent navigation services. Contact state or local autism family support organizations and ask about family groups for information and support.

Communication Needs

Autistic children may have unique communication needs and preferences, particularly in specific settings or times of the day. Some may struggle with social cues and nonverbal communication and understand more direct communication. For example, saying, "Take a seat" rather than "Please sit in this chair" might be interpreted as picking up the chair.

People with autism may require more explicit and concrete communication with preferences for visual supports, like pictures, written words, or sign language, as they may find visual information more comfortable to process than verbal information.[31] Visual supports break tasks into smaller steps, and create routines and schedules, with visual reminders of rules and expectations. One example of visual support is a first-then schedule to help your child understand the sequence of two events. It consists of two pictures or icons, with the first picture indicating an activity and the second representing a reward or preferred activity once the first task is finished. If your child uses a first-then schedule, remember to bring it to appointments and other outings to support your child during unfamiliar activities and transitions.

Some autistic people use augmentative and alternative communication (AAC) methods of communication other than speech, such as sign language, pictures, and text, to communicate and express themselves.[32] Nonspeaking autistics who cannot use speech to be understood need to be supported in using AAC to communicate. Common AAC devices and methods include communication boards, speech-generating devices, and picture-exchange communication systems. Parents may find a speech-language therapist or other professional specializing in autism to develop a communication plan that aligns with your child's needs and preferences. Check with your health insurance to find a speech-language therapist or experienced mental health professional.

Communication exists in many forms. Restricted repetitive behaviors (RRBs) can serve an important purpose for an autistic person, which we must try to understand before trying to stop the behaviors and find a replacement. A child who continually lines up toys may communicate a need for order, predictability, or comfort. For example, a preschool child paced back and forth as part of his RRBs. It was important to educate his preschool teacher that he should be allowed to walk around during circle time as he could pay attention that way and because it reduced his anxiety. Of course if such behaviors compromise the child's safety or the safety of others, alternative means of expressing their needs must be found.

There are evidence-based interventions that focus on social communication delays. Project ImPACT (PI) (Project-Impact.org) is supported by research based on developmental science. It is recognized as one of the most effective coaching programs for parents of young children with autism and related social communication delays. PI teaches parents strategies to help their children develop social, communication, imitation, and play skills during daily routines and activities.

Social Situations and Social Skills

Social Narratives

Social narratives are stories tailored to help autistic children understand social situations they may find challenging.[33] Social narratives aim to make these social situations less overwhelming and confusing by breaking them down into concrete steps and providing examples of responses. Customized social narratives can address a child's specific needs, using pictures, text, and even videos to illustrate social situations, such as visiting the dentist, how to sit at the dinner table, walking into school in the morning, and using a store dressing room to try on clothes. There are also resources for already-prepared stories.[34] When using a social narrative, you can read the story frequently leading up to the event and take it with you when you're out in the community.

Social Skills

Interventions emphasizing social skills development have found that these interventions produce modest positive effects.[35] Despite the focus on social skills training research, autistic individuals should never be forced to engage in social skills instruction. Social skill preferences and needs are personal and can vary from what society expects. Parents should consider their child's unique characteristics and personality rather than using a one-size-fits-all approach. For example, some people prefer time alone and don't want to be around many people, while others enjoy being the center of attention. Some people enjoy virtual interactions, while others are more comfortable in person. When autistic individuals are taught there is a "right" and "wrong" way to use social skills during social interactions, they may experience significant emotional distress because they feel they're pretending to be someone they're not. A phenomenon called *masking* or camouflaging refers to hiding or suppressing one's autistic traits or behaviors and imitating non-autistic individuals' social and communication skills, such as body language. By adapting to social norms and suppressing emotions, people try to appear more "normal" to navigate social situations that may be overwhelming or difficult. However, it can lead to emotional exhaustion and to mental health issues like anxiety, depression, and burnout.

Instead of forcing social skills norms, parents (and professionals) should strive to provide a person-centered environment, making self-advocacy the focus.[36] In talking with your child about social preferences, here are some questions that can help start the conversation:

1. How do you prefer to socialize with others?
2. What types of social activities make you feel comfortable?
3. What makes you feel anxious or uncomfortable in social situations?
4. Are there any specific social norms that you struggle with?
5. Do you prefer one-on-one conversations or group settings?
6. Are there certain topics or interests you feel more comfortable discussing in social situations?
7. Would you rather socialize with people who share similar interests as you or are different from you?
8. Do you prefer planned or spontaneous social events?
9. Do specific accommodations or strategies make social situations more comfortable for you?

10. Do you want to be open about your autism with others when socializing?

Bullying

The core characteristics of autism can unfortunately make a child more susceptible to bullying. At least half of all children/adolescents with ASD experience victimization.[37] Noah, who was in the fourth grade, had an affinity for facts about bottled water. He knew water sources, added ingredients, and strongly opposed certain bottled water brands. During lunch, he often criticized his peers for drinking water brands he didn't like. Sometimes, his peers would make fun of him, calling him "water boy."

A child may not know they are being bullied, misinterpreting the attention as friendship. Listen to how your child describes interactions with peers and consider asking probing questions that help you better judge the quality of the described friendships. If you have concerns, contact the school and let them know. Request that extra monitoring be provided during less supervised times of the day (e.g., lunch, recess). To monitor the situation, continue to discuss the identified peer or peer group with your child.

School System

Working closely with the school system is crucial to ensure your child's educational needs are appropriately met. Here are some strategies that you can employ:

1. Educate yourself: Thoroughly understand your child's rights, special education laws, and available services. This knowledge will empower you to advocate effectively for your child. Explore available resources and training opportunities to enhance your knowledge and skills regarding autism and special education.
2. Build open and positive communication: Develop a cooperative and respectful relationship with school staff. Regularly communicate with teachers, administrators, and support professionals to share information, ask questions, and address concerns.

3. Be actively involved: Attend parent-teacher meetings, individualized education program (IEP) meetings, and other school events. Show interest and actively participate in your child's education.
4. Understand your child's IEP: Familiarize yourself with the components of your child's IEP, including the goals, accommodations, and related services. Collaborate with the school team to set specific, measurable, achievable, relevant, and time-bound (SMART) goals for your child. Make sure these goals are individualized to address your child's unique needs and strengths. Ensure that the IEP team involves you in the decision-making process. Attend IEP meetings and actively participate in developing your child's educational plan. Provide input, express concerns, and collaborate with the team to make informed decisions.
5. Keep records: Maintain a documented record of your child's communication, assessments, and interventions. This record can provide evidence of progress or inform future decisions.
6. Request evaluations: If you believe your child requires additional assessments, request them in writing. Be sure to provide the school with any medical or professional evaluations you've obtained outside the school system.

Open communication, collaboration, and advocacy are essential when working with the school system. By actively engaging with the school and being an informed advocate for your child's needs, you can help ensure the best possible educational experience.

Accompanying Mental Health Concerns

Children and adolescents with ASD experience a range of medical and psychiatric disorders. The core characteristics of autism increase susceptibility to mental health disorders. Challenges with social communication can lead to frustration and withdrawal from social situations with high communication requirements: rigidity can lead to social anxiety; sensory differences can make one more susceptible to dysregulation; and stress is associated with transitions and unfamiliar social situations. Co-occurring mental health conditions are more prevalent in the autism population than in the general population: 28 percent suffer from attention-deficit hyperactivity disorder; 20 percent are diagnosed with anxiety disorders; 13 percent sleep–wake disorders; 12 percent disruptive disorders; 11 percent for depressive disorders; and 9 percent obsessive-compulsive.[38]

Anxiety

Evidence-based treatments for other disorders, such as cognitive-behavioral treatment (CBT) for anxiety, can be successfully modified and utilized for children with ASD experiencing anxiety.[39] CBT is a type of psychotherapy that focuses on helping individuals identify and change negative thoughts and behaviors contributing to psychological distress. CBT is based on the idea that our thoughts, emotions, and actions are interconnected and that we can improve our emotional well-being by changing our thoughts and behaviors. The therapy usually involves structured sessions where the therapist and client work together to set goals, identify thinking and behavior patterns, and develop strategies to address specific challenges. CBT can be modified and tailored to better suit individuals with autism by incorporating specific strategies and interventions, such as the following:

- Visual supports such as visual schedules, charts, and visual cues to enhance communication, understanding, and adherence to therapy goals. Talk to your child's therapist about particular child interests. If it's a specific character or person, that image can be incorporated into their visual support (e.g., cats).
- A structured approach to therapy can include providing clear instructions, setting explicit goals, and following a consistent routine that helps create a sense of security to reduce anxiety. When in therapy for anxiety, Addison's therapist used a visual timer to help her feel more at ease and less anxious about the length of the therapy session.
- Visual reinforcement systems, such as token boards or reward charts, visually represent progress, and reinforcements can help motivate individuals with autism and facilitate behavior change. Facing what scares you is hard! Talk to your child's therapist about therapy goals and reward them when they show effort or progress.
- Your child may experience sensory sensitivities or processing differences. Experienced therapists will consider sensory inputs and design therapy sessions to accommodate sensory needs, which

can improve engagement and reduce distress. Consider preparing a sensory bin with a few of your child's preferred sensory objects and give it to your child's therapist to use during their sessions. These familiar items may help your child feel more regulated during therapy sessions.

- More parent involvement. Your involvement in sessions and the implementation of interventions at home will generalize skills and promote ongoing progress. Plan to meet with your child's therapist to discuss therapy goals and the homework or practice that needs to be completed before the next session. Some therapists may provide a homework sheet to help you keep track of progress between sessions.

The modifications used in CBT for autism may vary depending on your child's unique strengths and challenges. An experienced therapist specializing in autism can tailor the therapy to meet child needs. The research shows that parent involvement and individual delivery (rather than a group setting) are optimal.[40]

Behavioral Disorders

Along with the core symptoms of autism, your child may exhibit broader behavioral problems, such as noncompliance, acting out, and explosiveness. Parent-child interaction therapy (PCIT) teaches parents various skills and techniques to enhance their parent-child relationship and effectively manage behavior. PCIT is considered an evidence-based treatment for young children with behavioral and emotional disorders.[41, 42] PCIT improves parent-child interactions, reduces challenging behaviors, and enhances family functioning. Some key features of PCIT include:

- Engaging in structured play sessions with your child while following their lead and allowing your child to make choices. Parents learn to provide labeled praises, reflections, and imitations to strengthen the parent-child bond. These skills are practiced at home during a five-minute daily special playtime. Reggie, a six-year-old with autism who loved trains, looked forward to special playtime with his mother, and the daily play helped her feel connected to her son.

- Setting effective limits and providing clear instructions to manage child behavior, including selective ignoring, effective command-giving, and time-out techniques.

Overall, PCIT can provide a comprehensive set of skills and strategies to promote positive parent-child interactions, improve child behavior, and develop a nurturing and supportive relationship. For more information about PCIT and to find a therapist in your area, please visit www.pcit.org.

Sleep Problems

Children with autism may have sleep issues, including trouble falling asleep and frequent nighttime awakenings, and the whole family may suffer negative effects as a result. Start by investigating environmental factors like the temperature of the bedroom, tags on sleepwear, or uncomfortable bedding. Bedtime routines are crucial for developing healthy sleep habits. Create a visual bedtime schedule, choose a realistic time for going to bed, give everyone in the family reminders, and be consistent. If your child is having trouble getting to sleep, you might need to create a sleep training plan. Depending on your situation, you can create this on your own; if you feel challenged or overwhelmed by this idea, seek guidance from a mental health professional. Sleep training plans are very individualized but often include details related to returning to your child's bedroom if they won't go to sleep or wake up in the night. When considering changes to the bedtime routine, check your schedule and try to pick a few days that are less demanding for you at home and work. Consider adjusting sleep routines during long weekends. When possible, seek support from a partner or another family member.

Medication

Although medication can't change the core features of ASD, up to 65 percent of autistic youth take medication,[43] which is 8 percent more than that of children with other DSM diagnoses.[44] Rates of polypharmacy (more than one medicine) are also significant.[45] The range of medications used are the following:

1. the antipsychotics, namely aripiprazole and risperidone. A significant proportion of children with ASD (20 percent) take these medications, and youth with autism respond better to antipsychotic medication for persistent irritability than children with other disorders do.[46, 47]
2. methylphenidate, atomoxetine, and alpha-agonists (ADHD medications) are the most frequently used, with 30 percent of children with ASD prescribed them.
3. selective serotonin reuptake inhibitor antidepressants for anxiety and depression are taken by 18 percent of children with ASD. These should be used with caution because of lower levels of effectiveness and high rate of adverse side effects, which may induce agitation.
4. mood stabilizers, the anticonvulsants.

The only medicines FDA-approved for ASD are risperidone and aripiprazole.[48] There is little compelling support for claims of effectiveness for most medications for children with ASD, except for using risperidone for aggression.[49]

ADOLESCENCE

During adolescence, your child may require various types of support to navigate the challenges and changes typically associated with this stage of development. Foremost, autistic adolescents should be encouraged and equipped to advocate for their needs. Work with your child to help them assertively communicate their preferences, accommodations, and boundaries, giving them a sense of control and autonomy in various settings.

Transition Planning

Adolescence involves preparation for the transition into adulthood. Planning for post-secondary education, employment, independent living, and self-care skills becomes essential. A personalized plan outlines the necessary steps, supports, and resources to facilitate a successful transition. Transition planning aims to ensure that individuals can achieve their goals and aspirations in various areas of life, including education, employment, independent living, and community participation. The process typically involves collaboration between individuals, their families, educators, and service providers.

The philosophy of supported decision-making (SDM) allows people with disabilities to get the help they need to make choices about their personal lives, health care, and/or finances.[50] This is in contrast to guardianship in which the right to make most or all life decisions is given to the court-appointed guardian. Self-determination is a key part of living an independent and fulfilling life. With SDM an autistic individual can exercise more self-determination and remain in charge of all life choices. When people make their own choices, they are more likely to live happier, fuller, and more independent lives. SDM ensures that people with disabilities have the right to remain self-determined and make life decisions. With SDM, an individual chooses one or more supporters for creating and communicating life decisions. Types of support provided may differ from person to person, but with SDM, people maintain their right to make choices about their lives. Mary is an autistic young adult who is employed and hopes to get her own apartment. She needed some support with finances and social life decisions but could make her own choices about medical care and employment. Her brother supports her in financial decisions, while her friend works with her for social life decisions.

Sexuality and Sex Education

Many people with autism do not receive adequate sex education. Additionally, they may have a more challenging time recognizing misinformation or understanding and applying what they have learned. Parents of adolescents with ASD are more likely than parents of non-ASD youth to report inappropriate sexual behavior and to have problems with privacy norms.[51] A typical example involves teens talking about their genitals and attempting to make conversation topics sexual in nature. Many curricula and trainings support teaching about healthy relationships, boundaries, consent, and sexual health and well-being.[52] Having a child with autism doesn't mean a person lacks interest in romance or has no sexual urges or desires. Talk with your child openly about their romantic interests and monitor what they search and look at online. To help your child avoid misinformation, you can find parent sex education resources online: https://asdsexed.org/category/resources/for-parents/.

Autistic youth may show more same-sex attraction due to heterosexist experiences, less sensitivity to social stigma, and perhaps difficulties finding opposite-sex partners.[53] Some resources for parenting gender-diverse teens are listed at the back of the book.

SUMMARY

Early diagnosis is crucial for timely intervention for ASD, which is typically based on parental concerns and observed developmental differences. Biological factors—genetic contributions, advanced parental age—play a role in development. Environmental and social factors may influence the timing of diagnosis but are not linked to ASD. A range of interventions are discussed with resources that can add further information. This chapter encourages acceptance and accommodation of neurodiversity, emphasizing the importance of understanding autism as part of an individual's identity and promoting inclusivity and support. Parents should learn about autistic culture by reading stories written by autistic people. Recommended books for parents are listed under Resources in the back of the book.

PART II

Internalizing Disorders

Chapter 3

Depressive Disorders, Self-Harm, and Suicidality

According to the *Diagnostic and Statistical Manual*, the depressive disorders that involve youth are:[1]

1. Major depressive disorder: at least a two-week period during which a person experiences at least five of the following symptoms nearly every day and most of the day:depressed mood; lack of interest/pleasure in activities; significant weight loss or gain; insomnia or sleeping too much; agitation or being slowed; fatigue/ loss of energy; worthlessness/guilt; lack of concentration; suicidal ideation; irritability.
2. Persistent depressive disorder: chronic, ongoing symptoms similar to, but less intense than, those of major depression.
3. Disruptive mood dysregulation, which is covered in chapter 7.

Depression in children is relatively rare, but in adolescence, new cases rise,[2] and depression is increasing among twelve- to seventeen-year-olds compared to every other age-group.[3] In the recent Youth Risk Behavior Survey,[4] more than 40 percent of high school students reported feeling persistently sad or hopeless. Suicide rates for this age-group increased over 50 percent between 2000 and 2022.[5] Overall, 22 percent of the nation's youth had seriously considered suicide, and 10 percent had attempted to do so.[6] In this chapter, depressive disorders are covered, along with associated features, self-harm and suicidal thoughts, the latter of which is a symptom of major depressive disorder.

The term *self-harm* is used in this chapter rather than the more official *non-suicidal self-injury*, which is defined as "intentional and non-socially acceptable behaviors intended to cause destruction or impairment of bodily tissues but only minor or moderate physical harm, performed without any conscious suicidal intention, self-directed, and used to reduce psychological distress."[7] The most common method is "cutting," followed by head banging, scratching, hitting, and burning.[8] Self-harm is not a diagnosis in the *DSM*, but depression and other diagnoses (PTSD has self-destructive acts as a symptom) are usually present with it.[9]

WHAT IS IT LIKE TO PARENT THIS CHILD?

What are signs you may have noticed about your child? He may not smile like he used to. She has lost her joie de vivre. They don't seem excited or look forward to things that once enthralled them. Some parents might feel annoyed with a child who seems like they're being difficult on purpose. If you struggle with depression, as well, it may make you feel worse to be around your child when they're like this. It's also downright scary to see a change come over your child. You're worried about them hurting themselves and what might happen. If you discover actual self-harm, it's very frightening, and you feel heartbroken that the precious child you birthed (or adopted) wants to harm themselves in this way.

WHY IS MY CHILD LIKE THIS?

Biological

Major depression tends to run in families, which supports, at least in part, a process of genetic transmission. Researchers understand major depressive disorder as "moderately" heritable.[10] The serotonin transporter gene is the most studied, and a shorter variation of this gene is believed to slow down the speed at which serotonin neurons can adapt to changes in environmental stress.[11]

Modifiable risk factors at the biological level involve a healthy diet and sleep.[12] Sleep seems to play a critical role in depression and suicidality. Teenagers reporting five or fewer hours per night were over 70 percent more likely to suffer from depression and almost 50 percent more likely to think about hurting themselves than those who slept eight hours nightly.[13] Three-quarters of teens don't receive the recommended eight to ten hours of sleep.

Depression in mothers is a particular risk factor for youth depression[14] for many reasons (note that paternal depression also plays a role, but there are far fewer studies on paternal depression). Genetic factors may be involved, given the heritability of depression. Maternal maltreatment history can play into their depression and then be transmitted to children.[15] Parenting may be affected by depression due to emotional unavailability, negative bias, and helplessness and inconsistency amid parenting challenges.[16] Parents may model depressive affect, thinking patterns, and behaviors that their children may imitate. For all these reasons, if you're depressed, please seek treatment and support.

Psychological

Increased vulnerability for depression may occur in adolescence because the capacity for personal reflection, abstract reasoning, and formal operational thought develops. That is, the development of cognitive ability brings with it the ability to think about the reasons for events in their lives. Teens may develop a depressive attributional style,[17] which attributes negative events to internal, stable, and global attributions: "I failed the test because I was stupid"; positive outcomes are ascribed to external, transient, and specific reasons: "I passed the test because it was easy." Adolescence is also when a future orientation develops, and they may feel hopeless about the future.[18] Hopelessness is a symptom of depression and a risk factor for self-harm.[19]

Rumination, the tendency to think about the whys of a situation on an endless loop without resolution, is implicated in depression. Coping strategies that are protective, in contrast, are the temporary use of distraction and problem-solving.

For self-harm, teens have identified some typical reasons for the behavior: (1) difficulty expressing an emotion; (2) a need to establish control over a situation that is experienced as uncontrollable; (3) distraction from a negative state, often self-loathing, worthlessness, or anger; (4) to punish themselves or others;[20] and (5) to see if anyone cared.[21]

Social Environment

As mentioned for other disorders in this book, a gene-environment interaction is most likely responsible for youth depression.[22] Environmental
factors include stressful life events, gender roles, peers and relationships, school, and cultural and societal influences. Table 3.1 shows the
risk factors that parents may be able to modify.

Stressful Life Events and Family Factors

We discuss family factors and adversity together, as stressful life events
often happen in the family context. Stressful life events[23] and childhood
maltreatment,[24] particularly sexual abuse,[25] are associated with depression. The greater the number of adverse life events, the greater the
youth's suicidal behavior in a review of twenty-eight studies.[26] Family
conflict is a risk factor for depression and self-harm and can trigger a
self-harm incident.[27] "Wanting to feel like somebody cared" is a reason
for self-harm.[28]

Often, a child presenting with depression will have an identifiable
event that triggered the depression, such as loss of a romantic relationship or friend group, maltreatment, moving, starting a new school,
parental divorce, etc. The place to start is to remove any stressful events
that make the child feel worse, such as bullying.

Cecilia brought in her six-year-old Grace for therapy because she
worried her daughter was depressed. When I met Grace, a serious and
unsmiling girl, she told me she was unhappy because her mother's
boyfriend planned to move in with them. Grace denied any abuse or
ill-treatment but said she didn't like him or how he treated her mother.
Grace said she had not revealed how she felt to her mother because her
mother was happy to have him in her life.

After receiving her permission to speak to her mother, I told Cecilia
that Grace did seem depressed and gave her the reason.

"She never told me that," Cecilia said.
"She knows you like him," I said.

Cecilia was adamant that they would proceed with his moving in
and decided not to bring Grace back for another session. The point of
this anecdote is your child might not have revealed what had sparked

or was maintaining their unhappiness because they knew you wouldn't be pleased.

Olivia had inadvertently started using her daughter Magda as a confidante for her marital problems with Magda's father. Although fourteen-year-old Magda was put in an uncomfortable position, part of her reveled in this important role. When Magda entered therapy, Olivia was coached to deal more directly with her marital problems and seek outside support from other family members, as she wasn't willing to go to therapy for herself. Because Magda might not like losing the special attention, Mom was also coached on other ways to spend time together that would boost their mood.

Gender

Another consistent finding is the greater risk for depression in girls and women that emerges in adolescence (about age thirteen) and persists throughout the life span. The gap between girls and boys seems to be widening.[29] Girls are also more likely to self-harm[30] and to attempt suicide.[31] Biological reasons for this gender disparity include reproductive hormonal development in girls—specifically estradiol, the primary female sex hormone, which influences the neurotransmitter and hormonal systems.[32] Increased stress in terms of stressful life events and, in particular, being bullied at age twelve was similar among girls and boys but seemed to have a stronger impact on predicting depression at age fourteen for girls than boys.[33]

Girls are more likely to use the coping strategy of rumination, which, as discussed, is problematic.[34] Girls are at greater risk of sexual abuse than boys, and experiencing abuse leads to risk for depression, self-harm, and suicide attempts.[35]

School and Peers

School failure[36] and a lack of connection to school are associated with suicidal ideation and suicide attempts.[37] Having supportive friends protects against depression[38], whereas bullying, including cyberbullying (being either a perpetrator or a victim), is associated with depression, with higher frequencies of bullying (physical, verbal, or relational) having a linear relationship to depression.[39] Peer conflict, rejection, isolation, and romantic disappointment[40] can trigger self-harm in vulnerable teens.

As parents, we're afraid of a contagion effect of depression or self-harm, or, God forbid, suicide attempts. Researchers found that rather than a "copycat" effect, people with preexisting vulnerabilities gravitate to those that appear similar to themselves, such as Goth or emo subgroups.[41]

Gender and Sexual Minorities

About 25 percent of today's teens identify as LGBTQ[42] and seem to have a much more fluid definition of both gender and sexual orientation than earlier generations had. I wouldn't overreact if your child tells you that they are LGBTQ or try to argue them out of it. You can explore with them the reasons for their conclusion. Many adults say that they recognized that they were LGBTQ at a young age. But some middle school youth have yet to be attracted to anyone and typically lack experience. They may need more time to sort out their feelings amid an emerging identity.

High school teens have a better sense of their sexual orientation and identification. If your child has told you they are LGBTQ at this stage, it's time to take it seriously. Ask about any bullying they're experiencing; if there is, you can coach your child on talking to appropriate officials and personnel. At that age, they don't want you to call the school for them. Remy and her husband refused to accept that their child was gay. They thought he was having a phase and would "get over it" if they pretended it didn't exist. This stance persisted despite the fact that he was now seventeen, and they had caught him in a sex act with a same-sex partner.

This discussion is all to say that LGBTQ youth report higher rates of depressive symptoms and disorder, suicidal ideation, behaviors, and self-harm,[43] likely due to the combined effects of fear of family and peer reactions to their coming out, bullying, and discrimination.[44] However, factors also protect against depression, including a positive LGBTQ identity, self-esteem, peer social support, connection to the school, and family support.[45] Therefore, you, as a parent, can provide some of these protective factors.

Table 3.1. What Parents Can Do About Modifiable Risk Factors for Depression

1. Offer healthy diet.
2. Don't allow young people to have their electronic devices with them all night as they often stay up on them rather than sleep. Have them checked in, blocked, or turn off the internet at night.
3. Since more screen time is associated with more depression, limit screen time.
4. If your child hasn't yet been given access to screens/devices, this is easier to implement, but having a rule about only using screens/devices in public spaces in the house; that may help with youth being in their rooms/in bed/isolating all day.
5. Show warmth and support even when teens seem to push you away. Try to empathize with struggles, with phrases like "That sounds very painful." "You were hurt." "You wanted someone to pay attention."
6. Improve parent-child communication so your child can come to you when feeling badly or in a crisis.
7. Balance monitoring and child autonomy.
8. Intervene as appropriate in any bullying or other precipitating factors for depression.
9. If your child comes out as LGBTQ, be supportive and accepting, even if religious or other beliefs say otherwise.
10. Treat any parental depression separately.
11. Get couples therapy for parental conflict.

Screen Time and Social Media Use

Teens report being on their phones "almost constantly" now, but emerging evidence links increased time spent on screens for leisure and entertainment with depression among both preadolescents[46] and adolescents.[47] Liu, Wu, and Yao (2016) found that the more screen time, the more distress suffered. Risk only decreased when it was fewer than two hours a day. This finding lends empirical support to the American Academy of Pediatrics guideline of limiting screen use to two hours a day, but for today's teens, this may pose an impossible goal.

IDENTIFICATION AND ASSESSMENT

The *DSM* criteria for major depressive disorder is slightly different in teens than it is for adults with irritability as a symptom.[48] Sullen crankiness can be part of adolescence, but if pervasive and long-lasting, irritability might signal a depressed mood. It's sometimes difficult to tell depression from normal adolescence, but if, over a period of a few weeks, you see your child isolating, negativistic, irritable, and critical, then it may be time to initiate a conversation: "I've noticed you seem sad lately. You're quiet and in your room a lot (or any of the other symptoms). What's going on?" or "I've noticed that small things are getting you down these days. What's going on with that?"

A recent client, age twenty-three, talked about being depressed since middle school. He had been unable to go to college or have employment since graduating high school. When we talked about the lack of recognition of his symptoms by his parents and teachers, he said that his father had mentioned once, "Are you depressed or something?" The gruff way his father asked this immediately caused my client to go on the defensive and deny it, and no one else attempted to intervene until he sought help as a young adult.

A child might also deny depression, perhaps because of embarrassment, shame, or fear of vulnerability, which are also part of depression. For instance, only about 50 percent of teens who self-harm will disclose; when they do, it's typically to a friend.[49] Unfortunately, friends don't always know what to do with that information and should be encouraged to tell parents or a school counselor. Teens who self-harmed described adverse reactions from parents, such as being ignored or dismissed, or angry, critical, and abusive responses.[50] Obviously, parents should take seriously their child's admission of depression and self-harm and restrain angry and critical responses, which are likely because they're scared. Show concern and support, and seek help.

Sometimes a child might confide something that seems minor, and you think, "They better get used to stuff like that because it happens all the time." The outward response is to offer empathy, however. The apparently trivial event is hitting them hard, has triggered something deeper, or touched on a core belief they have about themselves, such as "I am unlovable" or "I am worthless." As an example, Gloria's daughter, age fourteen, experienced a severe episode of depression after a long-term crush asked another girl to a school dance. Gloria's mother was responsive: "I can see why you'd be disappointed that he asked another girl to the dance. You thought you were going together. It feels like a betrayal."

Welcome tears as they indicate a release of emotions that have been pent up or blocked. Try not to show your surprise or shock, otherwise, they may feel ashamed for being babyish and uncool. Comfort them and let them cry. Don't offer tissues, as that implies to clean up and not express emotion (therapist tip).

If your child denies that anything is wrong and you have tried more than once to get a conversation going, but there still seem to be concerning depressive symptoms, I would err on the side of getting help. Depression that starts young is more likely to persist. It can also lead to substance abuse as prolonged pain begs for relief.

What to do if they reject help? Often, this reflexive rejection is a defense against intense vulnerability. Talking to someone outside the family about personal matters seems anathema to them. I would negotiate a stance which is particularly salient if they're not meeting age-appropriate expectations: "I'm concerned about how you're feeling. This is treatable, so you can get past this and feel like yourself again. If you can get out of bed on weekends and do your schoolwork, I'll know that things are all right, but if I still see that you're unhappy three weeks from now, I'll take that as a sign that more is needed. This is only because I care how you feel, and is in no way a punishment."

Some teens who have a perfectionistic mindset, which plays into both depression and anxiety, might balk at the mention of getting help because that would indicate they're not "perfect" and that something is wrong. In these cases, you can say: "I know you want to excel in everything you do. But we love you no matter what and are concerned that you're putting too much strain on yourself. If we have led you to believe that you must do all this for us, we'd much prefer you to be healthy and happy. It's not a weakness to talk to someone; it takes strength and courage."

If your teen continues to absolutely refuse, I suggest seeking help for yourself on how to get guidance and support. It's hard to live in an atmosphere of depression with a suffering teen who can often be sullen and irritable. If you're from an ethnic minority group, you may also suffer from increased fatigue and physical problems from caring for a teen with depression. Importantly, a therapist can advise you on how best to communicate with and help your child, and can make recommendations on their treatment.

PSYCHOSOCIAL INTERVENTION

Depression

Currently, most adolescents with depression have received past-year treatment.[51] Unfortunately, only a minority obtain treatment designed for depression or delivered from the mental health sector.[52] Therefore, I attempt in this chapter to guide you to the evidence-based therapies, which center on cognitive-behavioral treatment and interpersonal psychotherapy. The evidence for family therapy, play therapy, psychodynamic therapy, and supportive therapy, all of which are practiced widely, is "insufficient" to recommend these treatments, according to the 2022 Guideline Development Panel for the Treatment of Depressive Disorders.

Cognitive-Behavioral Treatment

Cognitive-behavioral treatment, which I'll abbreviate to CBT, is a present-focused treatment that leans on techniques derived from learning theory (operant conditioning, classical conditioning, cognitive learning, and modeling). For depression specifically, one representative treatment for teens, The Adolescent Coping with Depression course,[53] has the following typical components:

1. cognitive restructuring which involves:
   a. identifying negative thinking and beliefs, such as "This won't work out," "Just my luck," and "Everybody hates me"
   b. examining their validity, which is a specific element that teens find helpful in treatment[54]
   c. helping restructure the patterns into more realistic appraisals.
2. social skills training: how to make and maintain friendships
3. communication and social problem solving: how to share feelings and resolve conflict without alienating others
4. progressive relaxation training to ease stress and tension and to detach from unhelpful thinking patterns
5. structuring mood-boosting activities into daily life.

This treatment is short-term, delivered over fifteen or sixteen sessions, and is fully downloadable for clinicians (see Resources at the end of the book).

Behavioral activation is another cognitive-behavioral treatment for teens,[55] which helps individuals structure their daily life with tasks and pleasant activities to experience mastery and pleasure.[56] Behavioral activation is a good choice for teens that are sedentary and isolating.[57] Note that in any of the cognitive-behavioral treatments, family involvement might be important for recovery, particularly with children younger than twelve.[58]

Group treatment can be as effective as individual,[59] and, in my experience as a therapist, it's easier to get a whole group working on the structured material that is part of cognitive-behavioral therapy than it is individually. Unfortunately, groups are hard to find, and even more specifically, evidence-based group treatment.

Interpersonal Psychotherapy

Interpersonal psychotherapy (IPT) (IPT-A for adolescents) is a brief (twelve to sixteen sessions) intervention focusing on how current relationships have contributed to depression, with issues such as loss, isolation, abuse, conflict, and change in schools and neighborhoods.[60] The goals of IPT are to decrease depression and improve interpersonal functioning. Sessions are mostly individually with the child, though parents may be involved as appropriate. IPT-A has been effective in both individual and group formats.[61] The most recent comprehensive review of youth depression treatment found that interpersonal therapy outperformed CBT.[62] Interpersonal therapy is not as widely disseminated as CBT though, so CBT is generally more accessible. See the resources at the end of the book for more information.

Self-Harm and Suicidal Ideation/Attempts

The research supports dialectical behavior therapy (DBT) for teen self-harm and suicidal ideation.[63] DBT is an intensive intervention with multiple modalities—group; individual; family; phone check-ins; and supervision of therapists—for young people that are chronically self-harming. It originated for adults and has been adapted for adolescents (DBT-Adolescent).[64] Although it draws on the principles of learning and so is similar to cognitive-behavioral therapy,[65] DBT acknowledges some contradictions and traps that a teen may get stuck in, such as the challenge of balancing one's needs for both self-acceptance and change, and the acknowledgment that the teen needs to reduce stress, and self-harm might lead to negative effects in the long run. The latter validates the teen's need to relieve stress while helping her use DBT skills to reduce stress long-term. Treatment aims to help these teens withstand intense emotion and engage in functional, life-enhancing behaviors even when intense emotions are present.

Multiple family groups for two hours a week focus on the following coping skills: mindfulness; distress tolerance; emotion regulation; and interpersonal skills. See https://dialecticalbehaviortherapy.com/ for more details. Individual sessions focus on skill application to real-life situations. Telephone consultations with the therapist are available between sessions to reinforce therapeutic goals and deal with any crises.[66] This is a six-month- long commitment.

While many therapists advertise that they do DBT, you may want to choose a program that specializes in DBT with certified professionals. See the professional certification page where you can search by zip code (https://dbt-lbc.org/index.php?page=101163). DBT is more intense than some adolescents and their families might need, considering its multi-component nature and the length of treatment, and may disallow teens from participating in sports, recreation, socializing, and other activities that might help mood.

Firearm Availability

Part of intervention for depressed suicidal teens is to remove access to lethal means, namely firearms. If parents are gun owners, they should have any firearms locked away where the child cannot possibly get to them. If you have a teen with depression and/or who has talked about suicidality, they should not be around guns period, as nine out of ten times a suicide attempt with a gun will end in fatality. Alarmingly, teens who are depressed and suicidal say that they have greater access to guns than their lower-risk peers.[67]

MEDICATION

Antidepressants are currently prescribed to 10 percent of girls and 5 percent of boys[68] in the US adolescent population. The selective serotonin reuptake inhibitor (SSRI) fluoxetine (Prozac) is often the first-line treatment because it has been researched the most for youth with depression and consistently appears to offer benefit over taking a placebo pill.[69] Sertraline (Zoloft) has also received support for use in adolescents but not children. More recently, there has been limited support for escitalopram (Lexapro), the only other FDA-approved drug for adolescent depression, and nefazodone (Trazadone), the latter of which is prescribed when a child has insomnia. The SSRIs can increase risk of suicidal ideation,[70] so youth should attend regular (monthly at first and then every three months) monitoring sessions. If a child is in psychotherapy, the therapist can also monitor suicidal ideation. Having a relationship with the therapist means that your child might share information with that person rather than a doctor seen less frequently. The other advantage, of course, is that your child learns about triggers for depression and learns to prevent these and to cope if that is not possible. The research also supports the combination of Prozac and CBT as more effective than either alone.[71]

Antidepressants take weeks (four to six) to take effect. Your doctor will start your child on a small dose to start and see how they tolerate it. Unfortunately, medication involves a trial-and-error process. Side effects depend on the medication and your child's makeup. Some of them, such as headache, stomachache, and nausea, will likely pass as your child's system gets used to the medication. That's why it's important to start with a small dose and titrate (go up) slowly.

Now available are genome tests that can reveal which medications may be effective for a particular child. Some insurance companies cover these tests now, but your doctor has to order them to gain insurance approval.

Most antidepressants are taken in the morning with food because they are designed to activate mood. An exception is Trazadone, which is not an SSRI but an idiosyncratic antidepressant primarily used for sleep. Therefore, Trazadone should be taken a couple of hours before bedtime to take effect.

SUMMARY

Depressive disorders are serious when they arise in youth, and treatment is necessary so that teens develop resilience as they emerge into adulthood. Adolescence is a prime period to intervene when young brains and personalities are still malleable to change. Effective treatments are available, and resources have been provided at the end of the book so that concerned parents can find specialist therapists to provide treatments with research support.

Chapter 4

Anxiety and Obsessive-Compulsive Disorder

Fear and anxiety are part of being human and can be helpful in navigating potentially dangerous situations and preparing for tasks and responsibilities at hand. A diagnosable anxiety disorder, in contrast, involves intense, almost unbearable anxiety that persists as a pattern over an extended period, which interferes with functioning and meeting age-appropriate expectations.

Anxiety disorders are the most diagnosed disorder in youth, with almost 20 percent meeting criteria for at least one anxiety disorder. Seven disorders are diagnosable, but the most common for children are separation anxiety disorder and social anxiety.

Separation disorder involves excessive fear of being parted from an attachment figure for at least four weeks with three-plus symptoms: excessive distress; worry; reluctance/refusal to go places, sleep away, or be alone; nightmares involving separation; physical complaints, especially stomachache.

Social anxiety disorder is out-of-proportion fears in social situations persisting for six months, and causes clinically significant distress or impairment.

Obsessive-compulsive disorder falls under the classification of this chapter because it has a strong anxiety component. Obsession involves recurring, intrusive thoughts that cause distress, such as fear of germs. Children typically have little insight into the irrationality of these fears. Some obsessive thoughts include but are not limited to, an overfocus on bladder control, germs, accidents, fires, and other seeming catastrophes.

The compulsive behaviors that follow are repetitive actions done to reduce the stress of the obsessive thoughts or to prevent a dreaded event, such as washing hands to reduce the distress over ideas of germs. Compulsions to assuage those thoughts may include, but are not limited to, excessive bathroom-visiting, hair-pulling or skin picking, counting patterns, hand-washing, checking locks, and arranging items in specific ways.

CURRENT USAGE OF THE TERM

As of this writing, if you have teenagers or young adults, you might notice that the term *anxiety* is sometimes overused or misconstrued as a stand-in for other emotions, such as a more normalizing "stress." In other words, someone using the word *anxiety* may not have symptoms that rise to the level of a diagnosis. In almost all cases of overuse, I see the term *anxiety* as an excuse: "I can't do such and such because of my anxiety." Rest assured, I'm not endorsing anxiety as an excuse to escape. That flies in the face of the research-supported approach to anxiety. While children need to feel heard when they're in distress, we don't want to foster attention-seeking in this way inadvertently. This chapter explains the balancing act that a parent with a child diagnosed with an anxiety disorder or OCD requires.

WHY IS MY CHILD LIKE THIS?

A predisposition to anxiety is *genetically based* but modestly so, except for OCD, which is more heritable.[1] Other biological vulnerabilities for anxiety include physical illness, such as asthma or diabetes.[2] This association could be due to shared risk factors that contribute to mental and medical illness and the increased stress of managing a serious physical condition.

If you have more than one child, you know they come into the world with different temperaments. The following types of temperaments increase risk of anxiety (the good news is that they are protective against externalizing disorders, like ODD [chapter 7] and CD [chapter 8]):

- *Low self-directedness*: prefers to be given instructions rather than forging out independently. The child likes to be told what to do rather than initiating. If your child is like this, they may be obedient and don't cause problems in other ways, so they go under the radar.
- *Anxiety sensitivity*: quickly panicking in response to bodily symptoms, such as a faster heart rate or breathlessness
- *A tendency toward sensitivity and negativity*, such as fear, sadness, self-dissatisfaction, hostility, and worry
- *Harm avoidance and behavioral inhibition*: timidity, shyness, staying away from unfamiliar situations[3]
- *Fear of uncertainty/lack of control*[4]

Along with these tendencies are those toward perfectionism and other rigid standards that over-focus on a quantitative standard and detail rather than a holistic appraisal that can be flexible, depending on the circumstances.

Besides a biological predisposition, your child's environment may contribute to anxiety. Often a genetic or biological susceptibility is set off by environmental stress. This can be as simple as a specific event triggering the anxiety. A phobia for dogs may develop after a dog bite or simply observing an attack on someone else. Similarly, if parents excessively warn about danger, children can develop fears and worry. It's so hard as a parent to find the balance: to keep our children safe from real dangers without infecting them with anxiety about possible calamity.

People who experience anxiety usually want to escape from their fears and avoid them. Although it reduces anxiety, avoidance unfortunately reinforces a negative cycle. The good news is that you can help your child reverse the cycle and work toward, if not being anxiety-free, being able to manage anxiety in healthy ways. The counterpoint of avoidance is exposure, a component that will be a theme of this chapter.

Other Stress

Sometimes, no specific event conditions the fear, but a stressful or traumatic life transition, such as starting high school or college.[5] Kelly picked her hair to the point of creating bald patches on her scalp when she began a new school in third grade with much harder work. Rachel felt nauseous during her transition to a new high school, leading her to leave public places like church or family outings out of fear of throwing up. Like Rachel, youth with anxiety can't always put these feelings into words, especially when they have physical symptoms, such as nausea and stomach ache/upset.

Family

Parents, well-intentioned and without meaning to, may contribute to their children's anxious behavior. Nicole, age ten, worried nightly about having forgotten a homework assignment and couldn't sleep. Her mother joined in the worry, asking her to replay everything she remembered the teacher saying about the assignment. The continual questioning only exacerbated Nicole's anxiety. Nicole's mother was also overly critical and demanded perfection on Nicole's homework assignments, making her start over, for instance, if there were too many cross-outs or erasures on a page. The therapist coached Nicole's mother to broach her daughter's concerns with the teacher, thus sorting out the homework situation once and for all and allowing Nicole responsibility for her homework.

Gender

Beginning in adolescence, girls are more prone to anxiety disorder than males, which persists across the life span. The gender difference, not well understood, may relate to biological and hormonal factors and social factors, such as sexual abuse and social pressure.[6] In their teenage years, girls worry about popularity, being liked by others, and their relationships, which are not always within a young woman's direct control. You have likely seen the media reports about problematic cellphone and social media use and their association with increased anxiety, particularly for girls. The concern with social and relationship status may translate to increased distress when steady social media consumption is the norm.

WHAT IT'S LIKE TO PARENT THIS CHILD

A child suffering from anxiety may arouse feelings of irritation, frustration, sympathy, pity, anguish, and identification in parents.[7] It's easy to become annoyed at constant drama over something that doesn't make sense. You become frustrated when they don't listen to reason. Some parents will think the child is just after attention. It can be hard not to flare up with criticism or lash out in frustration. A mom describes her five-year-old: "He is scared of EVERYTHING. And it doesn't matter how much we coax, sweet talk, or explain that it isn't dangerous or going to hurt him. How do I help a child that won't listen to reason? I want to be calm, but when he disregards anything I say, I get upset."

Some parents can't stand to see their children in such distress, and that's why they give in to their children's panicky demands. Their hearts bleed for their children's anguish, and they can't tolerate their children's anxiety themselves. Fortunately, there are ways to handle your child's anxiety more therapeutically and with better results.

WHAT PARENTS *CAN* DO

Take Care of Your Anxiety

As mentioned, often anxiety is a family trait. If you're aware you suffer from anxiety, treat that separately from your child's treatment. Sensitive children, predisposed to anxiety, can pick up on your fears and learn to fret, question, and obsess. If you can model a flexible attitude that orients toward expressing feelings and problem-solving, you can help your child immensely.

Relax Rigid Standards

We all want our children to be safe and successful, but too much control and pressure on them can interact with underlying vulnerabilities to fuel anxiety in adulthood.[8] Several of my adult clients who suffer from anxiety have recalled that when they brought home a 97 percent on an assignment, their parents would ask, "What happened to the other 3 percent?"

Some parents require that their children earn all As. From being an instructor myself, I know professors vary in their standards and expectations, so a portion of grades are outside student control. If asked for a concrete answer, my advice is to request As and Bs; this is still a high standard but provides some breathing room and backs away from a "perfect" ideal. I have heard parents rationalize the pressure for high GPAs by saying their children must get into a "good" college. They buy into the notion that only specific pathways in life are worthwhile and follow a rigid prescription for success. In these cases, it is no wonder then that children adopt this prescription for themselves, and such rigidity can foster anxiety.

The National Center for Education Statistics reports that in 2022, the United States had over seven thousand four-year colleges. In other words, plenty of options are available beyond what some parents define as a "good" college, i.e., an Ivy League university with only a 7 percent acceptance rate and other similarly competitive institutions. In my son's graduating class, many students take advanced placement classes with over a 4.0 grade point with extracurricular activities added to the mix. Yet, many colleges reject these competitive applicants. In other words, an individual's performance is important, but so are societal factors like the economy, the pandemic, and birth rates. Understandably, we want to offer the wisdom and knowledge we have gained about education and employment. We might have some regrets about our choices and wish our children to fulfill some of these instead. Or we might dictate that our child should follow what we have done. Ultimately, however, each person's path is their own.

Avoid Enabling

A term called *accommodation*, which is like *enabling*, is easy for families to fall into. Accommodation means allowing your child to avoid triggers, like going into a public restroom, participating in compulsions (e.g., handwashing), and providing excessive reassurance. Troy, eight years old, freaks out about germs and begs his mother to wash her hands because of "germs." Troy's mother sees her child in such distress that she wonders what the big deal is about going along with him and washing her hands. She also orders for him in restaurants because she doesn't want to see him so upset.

Your intentions are good, no question about that, but unfortunately, you're perpetuating the anxiety.[9] In behavioral theory terms, when accommodation to child compulsions removes child distress, the child continues to believe that the compulsion is required to feel better.

Reassurance-seeking by the child is another trap parents of anxious children get caught in. A child may ask repeatedly, "Am I going to be okay?" When you duly respond with a cheery tone, "You're going to be fine! Don't worry!" that doesn't help either. It's counterintuitive, but providing reassurance does not help a child with an anxiety disorder.

So what do you say instead? First, you'll have to prepare your child that you're going to change your approach around reassurance-seeking. You'll have to put it in your own words, but the basic message involves realizing that you've inadvertently fed into the anxiety by trying to make your child feel better. Therefore, you'll no longer be available for reassurance because it only feeds the anxiety. However, you'll be there for support and to help them cope in other ways. Then, when the behavior comes up, remind your child of the previous agreement and any coping methods, such as distraction ("Let's play 'I Spy' like we talked about") or breathing techniques ("Let's practice four square breathing together"). In other words, you can assist in their tolerating the temporary discomfort of the anxiety for long-term gain.

Stay Even-Keeled

This is a tall order, I recognize. We're all human, and the anxiety can put tension on everyone in the family. Many parents will give in and be sympathetic to the anxiety and then have a meltdown another day over the same thing. To kids who have an aversion to uncertainty, you being unpredictable or erratic can make them feel more unsettled. If you have other children, you know that all kids aren't as sensitive. They're able to let things go easily. One of the biggest challenges with parenting is finding the balance: supporting your children without spoiling them; teaching them how to be aware and take care of themselves without scaring them about the hazards of the world; and cheering them on academically without becoming so demanding that it promotes their worry.[10]

Reinforce and Reward Children's Efforts

In my experience, children with anxiety are keenly responsive to reinforcement/reward plans, more so than children with behavior problems. So see if you can tie their efforts to special treats, even if it's just playing a game with you or screen time. Young and elementary-age children can earn a point each time they practice defeating the anxiety, which can be traded in for a reward at the end of the week.

Encourage Problem-Solving and Flexible Thinking

As parents, we're master problem solvers. We face so many situations a day that we have to become efficient about taking care of what needs to be done. As a result, we often reflexively give advice when our children express a concern. However, anxious kids need to bolster their self-efficacy, which is their sense that they can face and manage what comes up in their lives. If you can get them to approach a situation from several angles by a question or two, you have fostered some flexibility in their thinking. Here is a quick guide to steering a conversation in a productive direction when anxiety comes up in your child.

1. *Validate*, as simple as paraphrasing what they've said: "You're scared about going to school today." There may be tears in reaction to validation; this is a healthy way of discharging emotion.
2. *Inquire* in a curious rather than accusatory way about what underlies the concern. "What's going on?" (open-ended) or "What scares you about it?" Asking for specificity will help your child develop insight and articulate their concerns.

Mira, age twelve, woke up with a stomachache and didn't want to go to school, so her mother asked, "What worries you about today?"

Mira: Seeing Sarah. She wasn't nice to me at lunch yesterday. She's going talk to Enela and not me, and then I won't have anyone to talk to."

3. *Encourage problem-solving in your child*

Mom reframes her daughter's concerns into a problem she can solve: "So you're wondering who to talk to at lunch? What are your options?"

Mira: I could just stay home.

Mom: Okay, that's one option (smiles because that one won't happen).

Mira: I could talk to Claire instead. She usually likes to see me.

Mom: Ooh, I like that one! What else?

Mira: I could try to go up to Stephanie, but if she's with Enela, I probably won't.

Only when your child has run out of ideas should you ask permission about whether they'd like to hear *your* ideas. Of course, that also means if your child says *no*, you'll have to respect that. To conclude the problem-solving process, ask, "What ideas do you like? You know you can choose more than one," and help your child develop a plan.

NIGHTTIME FEARS

Many parents I've worked with admit to a pattern persisting for years of their children sleeping in their beds. As one mom said, "My daughter is scared of everything. I have to turn on all the lights in the house until bedtime. And she won't sleep by herself either. She says when she's brave enough. . . . " I'm not addressing the cases where parents choose to co-sleep and don't consider it a problem. I'm referring to families where the pattern disrupts parents' routines, and they desperately want their children to sleep in their rooms. Often, such parents have tried the basics already, such as making the child's room as appealing as possible, installing night lights, watching *Monsters, Inc.* together, etc.

When these strategies haven't worked, I've found that a behavioral approach is effective and doesn't have to be that deep. Some ways to set up a system that is as easy and as simple as possible for you to maintain involve the following:

1. Examine if your child sleeping in your room meets your needs. Is it a way to avoid sexual contact with your partner, for example, or because you're lonely? This examination of any potential benefits must be dealt with first.

2. Set a goal not too far from where your children are now in terms of staying in their rooms. If they are in your bed every night, then requiring them to be in their rooms each day of the week is asking

too much initially. For instance, a more reasonable goal to start might be three days a week when they stay in their rooms. As they can meet this target and earn rewards for a couple of weeks, you can adjust the goal to one more day at a time until they achieve success with that consistently.

3. Individualize a reward that will be enticing to your child.
4. Track where the child can see (on the refrigerator, their door, etc.) the points and stickers that can accumulate to the prize at the end of the week. The visual reminder will motivate your child. For young children, stickers can be incredibly reinforcing in themselves.
5. The hard part is escorting your child back to their room when they appear at your bedside in the middle of the night. At that time, remind them of what they have agreed on and the prize at the end of the week. It hurts to get out of bed when you're comfortable and in a deep sleep. They may escalate at your new boundary, and you might gently but firmly have to resist any pressure. Power through by reminding yourself that getting better sleep is worth the effort in the long run.

One day a snowstorm hit while my daughter's friend, aged six, was over for a playdate. Her mother could not get to us, so I knew Kay would have to stay the night. But she had severe anxiety about being away from her parents as she slept in their bed with them. After some talking from all of us, Kay agreed to stay, and we set her up with stuffed animals for comfort. She said if she woke up during the night and felt scared, she'd come into my room, to which I replied that if that happened, I'd walk her back to my daughter's room.

Obviously, since I wasn't the parent, I didn't have the emotional investment allowing me to follow through. This would be much harder for a parent to hear their kids cry and plead, which is heartbreaking. All you want to do is give in and make them feel better—and go back to bed yourself. But then they won't learn how to work through their anxieties or worries.

INTERVENTION

How do you know when your child needs treatment? Certain developmental stages bring particular fears, which are considered "normal." Babies cry when startled and exposed to strangers. Toddlers fear separation from caregivers. Typical school-age fears are the supernatural, physical well-being, and natural disasters. Adolescents have social and anxiety concerns, which are generally fleeting. But if they persist over time, cause great distress, and affect academic, social, and family functioning, then they should be addressed. Untreated anxiety can become chronic or recurrent (comes and goes).[11] A startling statistic is that in adulthood, the average number of years people suffered from anxiety before being treated was fourteen. The lesson is to be proactive in treating child anxiety.

Where to Seek Help

Start with your pediatrician. A medical exam to rule out health conditions is an important first step anyway to rule out any medical reasons for your child's complaints. Children's anxiety often presents as physical complaints, such as stomachache or nausea. Some children will be anxious to the point of throwing up, and then they develop anxiety about vomiting!

I suggest getting therapy rather than medication as a first-line treatment. Your pediatrician might be able to give you referrals to community practitioners they work with. Recent research has indicated that while office-based visits for youth anxiety have skyrocketed, increased treatment, especially with psychotherapy, has not.[12] Therefore, you may have to advocate for your child to be identified with anxiety and receive intervention.

Psychotherapy: Cognitive-Behavioral Therapy

Cognitive-behavioral therapy (CBT) has been evaluated more than any other therapeutic intervention type.[13] Table 4.1 lists the elements found in most CBT child anxiety protocols.

The central aspect of treatment for anxiety revolves around exposure, a process by which the child learns to face what they fear,[14] becoming used to tolerating the anxiety trigger until it's manageable. Don't worry, your provider will not throw your child into the "deep end." First, the provider will work with your child to construct a hierarchy of situations from least to most feared and then work through these in order, conquering more minor fears before the bigger ones in a process called *systematic desensitization*. The provider will also teach your child coping skills that she may need to practice, such as relaxation training and using helpful self-talk. The point of exposure is for your child to learn that the situation is not dangerous, and that, without avoidance, the anxiety will naturally dissipate.

Individual therapy with children for anxiety is effective.[15] However, you still have a role to play, more so with younger children,[16] but even with teenagers, you might have to encourage them to practice skills, such as deep breathing or exposure homework.[17] Sometimes parents may need additional assistance because of their own frustration and distress at watching their child go through anxiety. Since stressors and adverse circumstances may naturally play into anxiety, a clinician might also work with a parent about changing stressful circumstances in the child's life.

A greater demand for parents exists in the OCD treatment protocol, which similarly features coping and exposure. The additional piece is

Table 4.1. Components of CBT Treatment for Child Anxiety

Component	Description
Psychoeducation	Information about the nature of anxiety and how it can be controlled
Monitoring	Frequency and duration of symptoms and triggers
Cognitive Restructuring	Identifying, challenging, and changing maladaptive belief systems that contribute to anxiety, such as *"no one likes me"* and *"I have to be perfect to be loved."*
Relaxation Training	Mind-body exercises that help control physiological symptoms are taught as ways to cope and can be effective for anxiety on their own.Breathing control: deep breathing
	Progressive muscle relaxation: alternately tightening and relaxing certain muscle groups
	Mindfulness: cultivating a practice of accepting and detaching from thoughts instead of letting them become consuming
Exposure	Facing the fears with support and in small steps

that after a child is exposed to the anxiety-provoking trigger, the parent coaches them to refrain from avoiding the stimulus or engaging in the ritualistic behavior. Steel yourself for tears, begging, and tantrums. It's hard to keep patience and fortitude but strain for an optimistic tone: "Hey, come on, let's show this OCD who's boss!" Easier said than done, I understand, especially with OCD, where the obsessions seem so illogical. Have a replacement activity available so the focus is not all on what the child *can't* do. What's something pleasurable or absorbing for your child to focus on instead of the habit? In my experience, it would be difficult for a parent to undertake exposure and response prevention without professional support.

Finding Appropriate Treatment

CBT has been found very effective for children with anxiety, even at fourteen years after treatment. One challenge for accessing treatment is finding a qualified CBT therapist with a lot of clinical experience with youth anxiety. You can waste a lot of time and money on treatments that don't have a focus. Resources at the end of the book can help you find a qualified therapist.

School

The school may grant accommodations through a 504 or an IEP if the anxiety interferes with learning. See chapter 9 for how to work with the school to apply for a disability service for your child, and the resource https://anxietyintheclassroom.org. Specific to anxiety, one common accommodation in the school is to receive "breaks" when the child experiences anxiety. Unfortunately, this works against the research-based advice, which is for the sufferer to manage the situation and cope rather than avoid or leave. A better accommodation would perhaps be a counselor visit after class to debrief, and for the counselor to encourage and support the child's efforts to cope and to attend the next class. When you go for your meetings with the school, you can request this from the team. Also note an IEP for an "emotional disability," which can include anxiety, might warrant regular counseling in the school for your child. I would just be vigilant to make sure that the counseling involves the evidence-based methods outlined here.

Antidepressants

The *selective serotonin reuptake inhibitors* (SSRIs) and the *selective serotonin norepinephrine reuptake inhibitors* (SNRIs) were developed for the treatment of depression but might work better for youth anxiety than depression.[18] Serotonin and norepinephrine are neurochemicals (affecting the communication system between neurons in the brain). Still, the action of antidepressants is probably not as precise as sometimes described. It might have an impact on other neurochemicals in complex ways that are not well understood by the scientific community at this time.[19] Four types of SSRIs—fluoxetine (Prozac), fluvoxamine (Luvox), paroxetine (Paxil), and sertraline (Zoloft)—and one type of SNRI, venlafaxine (Effexor) show benefits over placebo pill for reducing anxiety in youth.[20] Medication is comparable to CBT in its effectiveness, and even more effective when offered together for anxiety.[21] For OCD, the research supports escitalopram (Lexapro), fluoxetine, and sertraline, which were found to be effective over fluvoxamine.[22] One concerning potential side effect of the SSRIs is the increased risk of suicidal thoughts in youth and young adults. Being in psychotherapy at the same time is a way to keep track of these symptoms and any other side effects.

In addition to the medications named here, providers use a variety of medicines off-label, meaning the FDA doesn't approve them for that condition. Gabapentin, a drug that is FDA-approved for restless legs syndrome, is often prescribed for anxiety, as is hydroxyzine, which is in the same class as Benadryl but stronger. The benzodiazepines, such as Xanax, are not typically offered for youth these days, although I have students report that some of their clients are given these for anxiety. At that stage in life, children need to be taught how to manage, perhaps with the help of antidepressants, rather than taking a sedative that has addictive potential.

Complementary and Alternative Medicines

Many parents prefer that their children receive a natural approach, such as vitamin and mineral supplements and CBD, rather than relying on medication. Parents should keep in mind, though, that most supplements, vitamins, and the like have not been properly tested.

SUMMARY

Anxiety disorders in children and adolescents not only cause child suffering, but they can also infect the whole family. Parents can play a crucial role in supporting their anxious children by caring for their own anxiety and avoiding accommodation to their child's fears. Instead, they should encourage problem-solving and flexible thinking and use positive reinforcement to reward their child's efforts in managing anxiety. When anxiety persists or significantly impacts a child's functioning, seeking professional help is recommended. Cognitive-behavioral therapy (CBT) is an evidence-based treatment for child anxiety, focusing on exposure to feared situations and developing coping skills. Overall, proactive and early intervention can help children learn to manage their stress effectively and recover.

Chapter 5

Eating Disorders

Eating and feeding disorders involve extreme changes in eating habits and body image, with 13 percent of adolescents meeting criteria for one of the following:[1]

Anorexia nervosa (AN), which involves an intense fear of gaining weight, resulting in severe underweight achieved through excessive restriction or purging.

Bulimia nervosa (BN), which involves consuming a large amount of food followed by purging behaviors or fasting to prevent weight gain.

Binge eating disorder (BED), which involves bingeing without compensatory measures.

Avoidant/restrictive food intake disorder (ARFID) is a newly recognized condition that includes low interest in food, avoidance due to the sensory aspects of certain foods, and fear of potential aftereffects of eating, such as vomiting. This condition is often associated with autism spectrum disorders (see chapter 2), and research is now only starting to coalesce, so it will not be a focus of this chapter.[2] The category *other specified feeding or eating disorders* (OSFED) covers those who do not meet full criteria for any one disorder, and most teens fit in this category. Another term you might have heard is orthorexia nervosa, an obsession with a fit and healthy lifestyle and distress if they can't adhere to the regimens they have set. Though part of the modern lexicon, orthorexia is not part of the *Diagnostic Manual*: a teen would be diagnosed with OSFED if orthorexia was the presentation. In this chapter, I discuss eating disorders generally as the field has accepted a "transdiagnostic" (across disorders) approach, highlighting shared symptoms and overlapping risk factors. Additionally, when eating disorders continue, they often morph into one presentation or another.[3]

WHY IS MY CHILD LIKE THIS?

Recall from the introduction no single cause exists for mental disorders, and a multitude of risk and protective factors give rise to disorder. With eating disorders, the current understanding is that a strong biological propensity exists but combines with environment and experiences.

Biological

When it comes to eating disorders, genes play a significant role; the onset of puberty impacts the genetic expression of eating disorders, especially in girls.[4] Therefore, girls between the ages of twelve and eighteen may be vulnerable if they have other risk factors. Early menstruation is a risk factor: girls at that age may feel shame and embarrassment; they also tend to be shorter and heavier because they stop growing earlier. They may also face attention from older males for which they are developmentally unprepared.

Being overweight is another risk factor.[5] Children are often teased for being overweight, and their self-concept may be affected. They may be put on diets by parents and medical professionals. Such restriction and deprivation may then lead to lack of restraint and bingeing.[6] Frightened by gaining weight, a child may then resort to restricting further or some compensation via purging or exercise, creating a vicious cycle.

Psychological

Temperament and psychological factors can also contribute to eating disorders.[7] Perfectionism,[8] negative emotions,[9] and trouble regulating emotions have all been linked to EDs. It's also likely that those struggling with an eating disorder are diagnosed with another mental health issue, like depression, anxiety, or OCD. It's thought these comorbidities arise from shared genetic vulnerabilities rather than one disorder leading to the other, except in cases where starvation might affect psychological functioning.

Social

You probably don't need to be told that some segments of society have an obsession with thinness. However, it's important to note that most people don't develop eating disorders from these pressures alone, even when there are other risk factors.

Families play a crucial role in transmitting societal mores and values. We recognize now that parents should stay away from all body, weight, diet, and exercise regime conversations around their children, including teasing children about "puppy fat" and making negative comments about their own or anyone else's bodies.[10] Anecdotally, some young women I counseled had fathers who would comment with disgust on overweight women in public.

Parents sometimes struggle to find the balance between protecting their children, keeping them safe from harm, and letting them make their own decisions and mistakes. Overprotectiveness has been linked to eating disorders. Some teens develop eating disorders as a way to erect boundaries that they're not able to set in healthier ways, often due to fear of loss of love and approval. Thus, eating disorders can be seen as a way to resolve contradictory tensions symbolically.

Youth with eating disorders have, unfortunately, a risk of trauma history or enduring stressful life events.[11, 12] By definition, these events are out of a child's control, and control is a key feature of eating disorders.

Youth with eating disorders often have social challenges. They can be very self-conscious (especially about weight and shape) to the point of meeting criteria for social anxiety. They may lack social support, as well as key social skills.

Social media exposure may contribute to eating disorders following exposure to images through social comparison and taking on the thin-fit ideal.[13] Additionally, male and female athletes participating in body/shape/weight-focused sports and activities, such as wrestling, cheerleading, gymnastics, and ballet, may experience additional risk.[14]

Although eating disorders are more prevalent among girls and women, boys and men can also have eating disorders. ARFID, for example, is more common in childhood in males.[15] Other demographic factors are that white adolescents are more prone to AN, and those from ethnic minority groups report more BED.[16] Unlike other conditions, high socioeconomic status doesn't protect against the development of eating disorders.[17] The common belief is that women and girls of middle and upper socioeconomic status may be more vulnerable due to increased demands for social compliance and perfectionism. However, the research doesn't support socioeconomic status as related to any eating disorders.[18]

HOW TO TALK TO YOUR CHILD

If you notice any eating disorder symptoms, please initiate a talk with your child. Start with an open-ended type of question said in a neutral tone: "Hey, what was going on when you were crying in the dressing room about your thighs?" Allow your child to answer rather than asking more questions, such as "Why are you doing this?" "What's wrong with you?" or answering for them (e.g., "We love our bodies, okay?").

The child with an eating disorder typically feels intense vulnerability and may have developed an eating disorder partly for protection and control. Understand that from their point of view, teens derive essential benefits from their eating disorder behaviors. Rituals and rigid rules around food restriction may reduce guilt, provide comfort, and help the client feel in control. For some teens, eating disorders give their lives structure and a sense of purpose.

Therefore, shining light on the eating disorder may elicit a defensive reaction. If you ask and they deny, accept that for now rather than arguing or exhorting. You won't find a way to argue them out of distorted thinking, and you might create too much negativity to approach it that way. You've opened the door for another conversation, and you can say, "I'm here if you need me." Hopefully, that will enable them to confide at another point. If they don't within two weeks or so and the ED symptoms continue, you can say something like: "I'm still concerned about how you see yourself and how you view and talk about your body. I'd like to schedule an appointment with the doctor to get you checked out."

If the doctor shares your concerns, they will refer your child for treatment. *Early diagnosis and intervention are key* as a much better prognosis exists for those who get treatment closer to the start of the illness when they've had less time for the eating disorder to become severe and entrenched.[19] A caution is that eating disorders from adolescence continue into young adulthood over 40 percent of the time.[20]

SCREENING AND ASSESSMENT

The pediatrician might have been the first to raise concerns about height and weight plots over time during a wellness visit. Generally, primary care providers and therapists are notorious for not recognizing and treating eating disorders, another reason parents should be aware of signs.

A medical exam will assess for any physical impact of the eating disorder. In addition to a routine check-up, labs and medical tests can establish whether there's amenorrhea (cessation of periods), bone density issues, heart arrhythmias, and electrolyte imbalances.[21]

From my experience working in a generalist practice with various client problems, I advise parents to seek specialist treatment. Eating disorders are complicated with unique dynamics, and a devoted treatment center can offer more parameters and clear expectations from the start, namely that weight gain will be necessary to avoid a more restrictive setting. A dedicated specialty in eating disorders means the availability of a multidisciplinary team of providers, including a psychotherapist, pediatrician, dietician, and possibly a child psychiatrist who should have experience treating children and adolescents with eating disorders.[22] Although pediatricians may suggest that your child see a dietician initially, this is not research-supported and is usually off-putting, especially for those with AN.

An in-depth assessment from a professional specialized in eating disorders will explore risk and protective factors and the frequency and duration of: body image concerns; eating patterns; weight control behaviors; binge eating; and compensatory behaviors.

Most people with ED also show other mental disorders. Care must be taken to ensure that the concurrent condition was present before and not the result of the eating disorder. For example, in AN, starvation may produce the depression, irritability, obsessiveness, and anxiety that are often present. Best practice is to treat AN symptoms first and then reassess as the child's eating disorder improves.[23]

INTERVENTION

Although treatment goals should be individualized, some standard priorities follow.[24] The first involves weight restoration and achieving medical stabilization (if applicable). A second is to reduce the number of binge eating and/or compensatory behavior episodes, as early response to these indicators is a good predictor of treatment outcome.[25] However, the amount of defensiveness and secrecy around ED behaviors means that a teen might find it easier to begin with goals that don't focus on weight gain. Please expect to be involved in treatment, not because you're to blame but because of children's developmental limitations, such as lack of insight and low motivation for gaining weight, when they perceive the eating disorder as providing benefits.

Treatment Setting

Outpatient is recommended as a first-line treatment for children and adolescents.[26] In *partial hospitalization,* clients spend six to ten hours a day between three to seven days a week and receive meals, group therapy, individual therapy, dietetic, and medication management.[27]

Hospitalization involves admission to a medical unit at a medical or psychiatric hospital that involves multidisciplinary services. Inpatient treatment is indicated with the following risk factors:[28]

1. serious physical complications (malnutrition, dehydration, electrolyte disturbances, cardiac dysrhythmia, arrested growth)
2. extremely low body weight
3. acute suicide risk
4. lack of available outpatient treatment
5. comorbid disorders that interfere with outpatient treatment (i.e., severe depression, OCD)
6. a need to be separated from the current living situation.

Residential treatment involves housing clients in a non-hospital-based setting for an extended period (averaging about eighty-three days) with meal support, an interdisciplinary team, and individual and group therapy.

Family-Based Treatment (FBT)

Much attention in the research literature for adolescents with eating disorders, particularly AN, has centered on the Maudsley model, developed by Dare and Eisler at London's Maudsley Hospital in the 1980s. In the Maudsley model, the underlying concept is that many of the teen's problems, such as anxiety, obsessiveness, and depression, are from the effects of starvation. Therefore, weight gain is essential so the teen can restore cognitive capacity and functioning and benefit from psychotherapy. While not to blame, the parents are now responsible for working together as a team to ensure that their child eats while the adolescent maintains control of other aspects of their life.[29] Treatment takes place over ten to twenty family sessions throughout six to twelve months.[30] According to the research, FBT appears to work better than individual therapy and is the only "well-established" treatment for AN.[31] FBT is less effective for youth with perseverative thinking (repetitive rumination, brooding, and worry) or obsessive-compulsive features and those from single-parent households.[32] FBT can be stressful for parents because they are to persevere when their child refuses to eat and to insist when their child becomes distressed. In FBT-BN, treatment is like FBT-AN, except for disrupting bingeing and purging behavior rather than weight restoration. Adolescents and their parents work together more collaboratively because a pattern of bingeing and purging is often upsetting to the teen, unlike those with AN who derive comfort from their symptoms.[33]

Psychodynamic Therapy

Psychodynamic therapy is generally concerned with early childhood influences on personality and, in a nondirective way, works on inner conflicts. The research on psychodynamic treatment for eating disorders is referred to by different names, including insight-oriented individual psychotherapy, adolescent-focused therapy, and ego-oriented individual therapy, with the aim of identifying the critical developmental, relational, or emotional challenges that adolescents avoid through their eating disorder and to help them manage these challenges in a more direct and functional way. Treatment spans a nine- to twelve-month period and includes several parent sessions. According to a literature review, individual psychodynamic treatment has been categorized as "the second-best evidence-based approach" for AN after Maudsley family-based therapy.[34]

CBT

CBT for eating disorders is transdiagnostic with the recognition that the eating disorders have similar and overlapping risks and features.[35] CBT aims to improve coping, problem-solving, and social functioning. It involves self-monitoring of eating, what was eaten (not counting calories), when and where, as well as triggers. Along with a nutritionist-approved meal plan of three meals with two or three planned snacks, the parent monitors the child closely during and after meals. Over time, the youth has more independence around meals as they demonstrate that they're not bingeing and purging. Weekly weight is monitored.

CBT strategies help identify triggers for binge eating and purging and strategies to cope more effectively and to problem solve. Distraction is one tool, as is identifying and using replacement behaviors and enlisting support people to get through urges. The therapist also helps the client identify thoughts related to the ED, such as, "If I don't throw up, I'll get fat," and how thoughts, feelings, and behaviors are connected. The therapist teaches the client to challenge and change maladaptive thoughts. For example, a teen may say, "I'm so fat." This statement can be changed to a more helpful "The way I look doesn't determine my value as a person." The therapist will help the teen determine which peers are positive influences and work to increase supportive and positive interactions. The teen also identifies peers for whom continued association would harm recovery. They learn to problem-solve strategies to cease and navigate those relationships and how to avoid risky situations.

Medication

Evidence guidelines caution against medication for adolescents with eating disorders, but most teens are prescribed at least one drug, no matter the type of eating disorder.[36] For AN, the SSRIs (see chapter 3) are prescribed for comorbid conditions, such as depression, anxiety, and OCD, but only after the teen gains sufficient weight. If the child is underweight, low serotonin reserves are available, which hinders the potential effectiveness of the medication.[37] Fluoxetine (Prozac) is not FDA-approved for adolescents with BN, although it has approval for adults with the same condition and children and adolescents for depression and OCD.

Atypical antipsychotics (olanzapine and risperidone, typically) have been studied with adolescents with AN more often than antidepressants, but clear evidence of their efficacy is lacking.[38] Therefore, antipsychotics should only be used when comorbid psychiatric conditions exist alongside the eating disorder or to manage severe behavioral agitation temporarily when nothing else has worked.[39]

Promote Non-Weight-Related Interests and Activities

At the same time as you seek treatment, reinforce any other interests— a hobby, art, recreational sport, or competitive activity—as long as it doesn't encourage the ED. The ED is very consuming and absorbing. If your child can find other ways to sublimate, channel, and cope, they may reduce its hold. Even if it's an interest you've rejected before because of cost, such as skiing/snowboarding or expensive lessons, you may want to revisit what has piqued your child's interest, as it will be healthier and less costly in the long run than treating an eating disorder.

SUMMARY

Teens, especially girls, may be more at risk for eating disorder pathology, given the potentially harmful effects of social media, including unrealistic images, fetishization of fitness and health, and pro–eating disorder websites. Reducing social media consumption (limiting hours available) and promoting other interests will be critical. Parents must also curb their obsessions with diet, exercise, and their bodies to prevent risk. The recommendation is to identify and treat eating disorders when they first appear, as treatment is much more effective then, and to prevent the eating disorder from continuing and progressing.

PART III

Stress- and Trauma-Related Disorders

Chapter 6

Post-Traumatic Stress Disorder

Recall from the Introduction that the *Diagnostic Manual* generally assumes an individual rather than environmental causation. Still, the disorders in this chapter are thought to arise because of trauma or other adverse events that occurred to the child. Most of this chapter centers on *post-traumatic stress disorder*, but I also cover *attachment-based disorders* and *adjustment disorders*.

PTSD

The word *trauma* is often overused now in conversation, meant to convey something difficult. Still, for diagnosis, trauma has a narrow definition: a serious event beyond the bounds of everyday human experience, such as violence or witnessing violence, accidents, abuse, neglect, and abandonment. Certain types of traumatic events may also predispose a person to PTSD, such as war-related events (including refugee and immigration status), criminal victimization, and exposure to natural disasters. A child with PTSD develops symptoms in four categories:[1]

The first is *intrusion*, meaning a child reexperiences or replays the traumatic event. Children struggle to put their feelings into words and, depending on their cognitive level, cannot identify what they're thinking, as "thinking about thinking" is a meta-cognitive skill that children typically don't develop until adolescence. As a result, you won't often have access to how much a child replays the traumatic event since they can't articulate their inner experience well. Very young children might replay specific themes over and over again. My first child client was a three-year-old who had lived with neglect and was placed in foster care.

With dolls, she often reenacted a scene where her mother's boyfriend had been violent with her mother, and the police came. Other ways the criterion of intrusion comes up is through nightmares, which may evoke the same sense of powerlessness and fear, or being triggered by events associated with the trauma. Mona, age fourteen, experienced a boy sexually touching her on a bus and then became anxious about riding in buses.

The second symptom profile for PTSD is *avoidance*. The child tries to protect herself from how bad she feels by avoiding any triggers or reminders, including talking about it. Troy, a ten-year-old, wasn't compliant with taking a shower one night, and his father became enraged and had a stroke in front of Troy. Troy avoided showers after that, linking in his mind the shower that night and his father's stroke.

Negative mood and beliefs about the self, world, and others are also part of the symptom profile. These symptoms look like depression, and, indeed, depression, more so than PTSD, is a common outcome of trauma.[2]

The last part of the symptom profile is *increased arousal*, which involves symptoms of hypervigilance, insomnia, an inability to concentrate, an elevated startle response, irritability/anger, and self-destructive acts. Although anxiety appears in these symptoms, and the *Diagnostic Manual* used to group PTSD with other anxiety disorders, there can also be an angry/explosive presentation of PTSD, which may overlap with the conditions explored in chapter 7. Note, in addition, that "self-destructive acts" could include the self-harm that was explored in chapter 3.

Dissociation is a way that some children cope with trauma in which they "space out" or become removed from an event so frightening and uncontrollable that they feel like they are looking down or are at a distance from what's happening to them. Dissociation serves as a coping strategy to get through an intolerable event. However, it comes at a cost, as the event and its associations aren't processed, and dissociation may become a habitual way of coping. It's hard to tell when a child is dissociating because they usually can't describe it, and it may present as daydreaming or being "out of it." In the diagnostic criteria, dissociation is a subtype of the PTSD diagnosis. Dissociation should be treated if present so kids can integrate their experiences and not carry this forward as a coping mechanism.

You may have heard of the term *complex PTSD*.[3] This diagnosis doesn't exist in the US diagnostic system. However, it is in the World Health Organization International Classification of Diseases, the diagnostic system for Europe and much of the world.[4] Generally, complex PTSD involves a reaction to sustained, repeated, or multiple traumas that involve the PTSD symptoms described above, along with severe emotional dysregulation.

Prevalence

For youth, the chance of being diagnosed with PTSD is, thankfully, relatively rare. About two-thirds of youth undergo traumatic events, unfortunately,[5] but only a minority end up meeting criteria for PTSD. The overall rate of PTSD in preschoolers is 22 percent,[6] in children is 16 percent,[7] and in adolescents 5 percent.[8] The younger the child, the more susceptible.

Why Does a Child Develop PTSD?

At the heart of the development of PTSD lies a trauma, an environmental event to which the individual has been subjected, and features of the trauma event—severity, degree of exposure to the trauma (intensity, duration, and frequency), and the sense of perceived danger[9]—connect to the extent of adjustment.

Biological

The extent to which biological processes are risk influences for PTSD or result from the child's experience of trauma is unknown, i.e., the trauma creating dysregulation or impairment in brain functions. People with PTSD tend to have abnormal levels of key hormones (cortisol) in their response to stress.[10] As discussed in chapter 3, having a shorter version of the serotonin transporter gene appears to increase one's risk for depression, as well as PTSD, after exposure to extremely stressful situations.[11] This same gene variant increases the activation of an emotion control center in the brain known as the amygdala.

Psychological

The main theory about PTSD is like that of the anxiety disorders (see chapter 4), in which a child becomes conditioned to cues associated with the trauma and develops anxiety as a result.[12] Neutral cues, like riding a bus in the example of Mona, may become frightening and activating in themselves. Many kids will then avoid the once-neutral stimulus—people, places, and things that remind them of the trauma—which sets up a negative cycle of continued anxiety and avoidance.

Social

Research has identified several risk and protective factors for the development of PTSD. A secure parent-child attachment and family support more generally is protective.[13] For adolescents, prior trauma exposure relates to the development of PTSD in the face of another event. For preschoolers, interpersonal trauma is linked to greater risk.[14] For youth, living in an adverse family environment, particularly not with both biological parents, may add to the risk of developing PTSD after trauma. If you suffer from PTSD or have suffered a traumatic event in childhood,[15, 16] your child also may show increased risk. The precise mechanisms of how this works are unknown but could involve genetic predisposition, exposure to the same traumatic event (e.g., a car accident), and/or that PTSD negatively impacts parenting.

What Parents *Can* Do

Avoid Potentially Adverse Circumstances

Trauma is often experienced as uncontrollable. Obviously, and as much as we would all like to as parents, we can't shield our children from the misfortunes and accidents of life. As you're already aware, a child's circumstances can be traumatizing even if they don't directly experience events. I had one client who suffered from severe anxiety and depression and feared other men. He revealed a stepfather who was verbally and physically abusive of his mother. My client hid in his room to avoid bringing the abuse onto himself. Obviously, most parents are doing the best with what they have, but as much as possible, protect your child from potentially harmful circumstances, such as unvetted babysitters, abusive partners, access to guns, unstable living situations, and so forth.

If You Suffer from a Trauma Reaction, Seek Support

The trauma area for which I have the most expertise is sexual abuse. In that work, I've met many girls whose mothers revealed that they, too, had been sexually abused. Sometimes these disclosures happened for the first time, meaning that the mothers had not shared this experience with anyone before their child was part of a child abuse investigation. If you have your own areas of trauma, you might feel motivated to address them. The potential benefits to your child may include preventing future negative events occurring to them and to avoid them taking up your vulnerabilities in a process of intergenerational transmission. Many parents wouldn't necessarily seek treatment for themselves, but they might if they realized that there are both direct and indirect benefits to children when their parents have reduced depression and other symptoms.

Allow Your Child to Discuss the Event

I don't know how many times I've heard parents tell me they just want their children to forget what happened to them, so they don't want to talk about the traumatic event with their child. There are other reasons why parents might not want to discuss the trauma: guilt for not protecting the child and/or it's activating or upsetting to the parent. Some parents worry about not saying the right thing. In these cases, I advise answering children's questions about the event, e.g., "What's going to happen to Grandpa next?" You can also reflect their concerns. For instance, if a child says, "I don't know how we're going to have enough money without (stepfather) around," you can reassure them that those are adult concerns that you will grapple with and, ultimately, resolve.

A natural response to an adverse event is to try to make sense of it, which might involve children taking ownership for the event; in other words, they blame themselves. For example, a child might say, "I should have stayed in my room when I was alone in the house with him." Or "I shouldn't have walked that way home from school." People prefer to blame themselves for what has happened because then, in their minds, they at least have some control over the event. If a child does self-blaming, hear them out and see if you can reflect their perceptions: "You've been thinking a lot about why this happened, and you're trying to find reasons why." Then you can offer some reassurance that most of us do this and that they were not responsible for the traumatic event.

Children are also attuned to your signals about being willing to talk. We can often catch people's vibe about safe subjects and what is allowable to speak about. You might have to bring it out in the open to ensure that your child can discuss this topic: "How are you feeling now about what happened? What are your thoughts? Do you have any questions? I want you to know that you can come to me."

Assessment and Intervention

To be diagnosed with PTSD, a child has to experience symptoms for over six weeks, so the recommendation is that a provider, possibly the pediatrician, screen about three to six months following a traumatic event.[17] PTSD requires careful differential diagnosis as other disorders may be more appropriate, share overlapping symptoms, or are co-occurring. If you seek treatment for your child, you are better off looking into more specialized interventions for trauma, which are described below.

Trauma-Focused Cognitive Behavioral Therapy

Trauma-focused cognitive behavioral therapy has the most research support at this time. The components involve a focus on traumatic memories and their meaning.[18]

P: psychoeducation and parenting skills
R: relaxation training
A: affective expression and regulation, how to label and talk about feelings
C: cognitive coping (realistic and helpful self-talk)
T: exposure to the memories of the trauma through some kind of narrative development (going into the details of what happened, their feelings and interpretations at the time and currently)
I: in vivo exposure, meaning if there are cues that are associated with the event, the child learns not to avoid but to face and manage them
C: conjoint parent/child sessions or individual parent sessions
E: enhancing safety/future development

Exposure, meaning direct discussion of memories of the trauma, as well as talking about any cues associated with the trauma, is the central concept of this type of treatment. A therapist working from this framework will help develop a hierarchical list of aspects of the feared situation in rough order from least to most anxiety-producing. They will work through them in this order so that your child can gain some mastery over his fears one at a time. The therapist teaches ways to cope with the anxiety: relaxation training and breathing control, and ensuring self-talk is calming and encouraging. The therapist helps the child overcome the tendency of avoiding discussion of the trauma, which is thought to prevent the child from integrating the trauma and prolong the stress reaction.

Depending on the age of the child, cognitively oriented interventions may also be part of treatment. The therapist will elicit any problematic beliefs, self-blame, frustrating attempts to mentally "undo" the traumatic event, lack of safety, inability to trust, powerlessness, and loss of control. The process for adjusting these beliefs occurs in steps: the first is to identify the beliefs; then to challenge those that are inaccurate or unhelpful ("It's my fault this happened."); and finally, replace them with more helpful thoughts ("It's not my fault. I am a good person.").

Although much of the treatment will be done individually with the child, you will also play a role and attend some parent-child and parent-only sessions. Additionally, you may have to encourage your child to do any "homework" that is assigned, which usually has to do with extending the exposure exercises from one of the sessions. One difficulty that parents and children sometimes have with this type of treatment is that they find the exposure piece of the therapy distressing. Part of the syndrome of PTSD is avoidance, which means that the trauma and its associations and aftermath aren't integrated and remain out of conscious awareness; hence, the syndrome continues. However, the treatment technique of exposure demands that child clients not avoid what has been distressing. Again, this is done gradually as the child becomes comfortable, but children often resist doing it.

Keep in mind that the research has indicated that children benefit from this treatment over control groups and usual care regarding PTSD symptoms, depression, and anxiety.[19, 20] One area that remains untouched, however, is avoidance of cues despite the focus of the treatment. Acting in an adjunctive role, parents also find their depression, emotional distress, and PTSD reduced from their children going through this treatment.[21] Reducing depression relates to how well the child benefits from treatment. A version of this treatment based in the school for children who have experienced trauma (not necessarily diagnosed with PTSD) is called cognitive behavioral intervention for trauma in schools (https://traumaawareschools.org/index.php/learn-more-cbits/).

Play therapy is popular among community therapists for child PTSD, though little research has been done to support this widespread practice.[22] However, it might be helpful for very young children (preschoolers and early elementary age); one that has been developed and has received some testing is child-centered play therapy, delivered individually with parent meetings every three to five child sessions and in groups in school settings.[23]

Eye Movement Desensitization and Reprocessing

Another treatment that has received research support is Eye Movement Desensitization and Reprocessing (EMDR), which uses a client's eye movements (or other alternating bilateral sensory input such as noises, taps, or colors) to process traumatic memories. Francine Shapiro, its creator, has outlined the method in a book and created an international training program.[24] An EMDR therapist asks clients to keep a traumatic memory in their minds as the clinician elicits eye movements. There is also a cognitive component to EMDR, as the client is asked to identify and rate negative cognitions associated with the event to decrease belief in the negative cognition. Various mechanisms have been put forth to explain how EMDR works with no definitive conclusions.[25] Although fewer studies on EMDR have been conducted than on trauma-focused CBT, in synthesizing all the studies, researchers found that the two treatments had similar effectiveness for reducing post-traumatic and anxiety symptoms.[26] Considered an advantage for some, EMDR doesn't require a child to recount details of the event but focuses more on beliefs that may have evolved from the experience, such as those involving safety, self-blame, powerlessness, and helplessness.

Medication

The FDA has not approved any medications for PTSD in youth, although most youth with PTSD receive antidepressants.[27] A significant proportion receive antipsychotics, which are associated with serious side effects. Seven percent are prescribed benzodiazepines, which are related to risk of dependence. Medication use is more common among older youth with other health and mental health disorders in the southern United States, where there are more rural poverty areas and fewer psychosocial treatment providers.

ATTACHMENT DISORDERS

Another set of disorders in this grouping of the American Psychiatric Association diagnostic manual is *attachment disorders*.[28] Similar to PTSD, a child with an attachment disorder has experienced a major disruption of caregiving, severe maltreatment, and/or abandonment. If a child is adopted over eighteen months old, they may struggle with attachment difficulties. Children who've suffered these extreme circumstances might meet criteria for two different types of reactions. The first is *reactive attachment disorder* in which the child is withdrawn from caregivers, doesn't seek or seem to obtain comfort, and shows other social and/or emotional disturbances, such as explosive tantrums. The other is *disinhibited social engagement disorder*, which has the opposite profile: a child approaches strangers and unfamiliar adults in an overly familiar way, without regard for safety. The other similar feature of both attachment disorders is the other social and emotional disturbances, such as explosiveness, oppositionality, and tantrums.[29]

Parenting children with attachment disorders is challenging; due to their history of instability and abandonment, they sadly re-create these patterns. Because they don't respond to affection and support and seem compelled to drive away people with their behaviors (explosiveness, verbal abuse, physical aggression), they are set up for more attachment failures, and the negative cycle continues. Parenting a child with attachment disorders requires a lot of support because a child like this may, at times, act in ways that make you feel like they hate you. It's hard to maintain warmth, attunement, and consistency in the face of these reactions, which is what the child needs. For very young children, birth to five years, an intervention called child-parent psychotherapy has support in randomized, controlled trials for improving the attachment relationship between parent and child.[30] For the explosiveness and tantrums, the interventions described in chapter 7 on ODD/DMDD might prove useful, particularly parent-child interaction training, which focuses on developing parent-child attachment and behavioral management. For adolescents suffering from PTSD, there is a group program called CONNECT for parents.[31] While the United States often leads on child and adolescent mental health research, CONNECT is only starting to be studied here. Countries as diverse as Sweden, the U.K., Italy, Canada, Mexico, South Africa, and Australia have used this model to improve adolescent attachment problems and aggressiveness to good effect. One bonus is that the intervention is for parents, as it can be difficult to engage an adolescent struggling with attachment issues in therapy.

ADJUSTMENT DISORDERS

Most therapists in outpatient settings will diagnose children with adjustment disorders, which have to do with a child reaction (emotional and/or behavioral) to a stressful life event within three months. Additionally, the reaction doesn't extend beyond six months of resolution of the stressor. Providers often use such a diagnosis because they are cautious about potential stigmatization and having a third-party payer record of a more serious disorder. In my experience in outpatient settings, the assignation of an adjustment disorder is usually easy to justify; most people have had a recent event that has stimulated their seeking out therapy.

The *DSM*-5 lists six different types of adjustment disorders:[32]

1. with depressed mood
2. with anxiety
3. with mixed anxiety and depressed mood
4. with disturbance of conduct
5. mixed disturbance of conduct and mood
6. unspecified (symptoms vary from the other types).

The main reason for an adjustment disorder is a stressful life circumstance, so hopefully you can help your child resolve the situation. Depending on what type of adjustment disorder, the evidence-based treatment associated with the problem might also be helpful. For instance, if a child is diagnosed with adjustment disorder with *anxiety*, techniques from CBT for anxiety can be used so that the child attains a better level of functioning.

SUMMARY

This chapter covers disorders that result from traumatic events and other adversities, with a primary focus on post-traumatic stress disorder (PTSD) but also attachment-based disorders and adjustment disorders. For PTSD, parents can support their children by avoiding adverse circumstances, seeking help for their own trauma reactions, and encouraging open discussions about the traumatic event. Interventions like trauma-focused cognitive behavioral therapy (TF-CBT) or eye movement desensitization and reprocessing (EMDR) can be beneficial.

Attachment disorders stem from severe maltreatment and can be present in adopted or foster children and require specialized parenting support. Adjustment disorders, triggered by stressful life events, are commonly diagnosed in outpatient settings. The focus is on changing stressful circumstances for the child and helping them cope and adjust.

PART IV

Externalizing Disorders

Chapter 7

Oppositional Defiant Disorder and Disruptive Mood Dysregulation Disorder

Some of the most challenging behaviors to deal with are tantrums and explosiveness. Oppositional defiant disorder (ODD) and disruptive mood dysregulation disorder (DMDD) are the diagnoses that chiefly feature these patterns. The *Diagnostic Manual* organizes them into separate chapters: ODD is in the *disruptive behavior disorders* chapter, and DMDD is a *depressive disorder.*[1] DMDD was formulated to address the overdiagnosis of bipolar disorder in youth. See the Introduction for a brief history, but basically children received the bipolar disorder diagnosis when they displayed a symptom profile of extreme negative mood and irritability, rather than the criteria in the DSM. If your child has been diagnosed with bipolar disorder, then the information in this chapter about DMDD is likely still relevant.

ODD and DMDD feature anger/irritability, temper tantrums, argumentativeness, and opposition. ODD involves a profile of angry/irritable, defiant/oppositional, and vindictive behavior over six months. ODD is important to treat when the child is young since almost half (40 percent) of those diagnosed go on to develop the more severe conduct disorder (CD),[2] which features aggression, violation of rules, and deceitfulness. Chapter 8 covers CD, along with substance use disorders. Both typically involve teenagers (although CD can be "child onset") and usually go hand in hand, sometimes involving the legal system. This chapter primarily focuses on younger children (preschool to middle school).

DMDD features irritability and a tendency toward anger and temper outbursts.[3] Irritability is considered a transdiagnostic symptom, which means that it's present in different disorders and seems to be a factor associated with long-term impairment.[4]

ODD is differentiated from disruptive mood dysregulation disorder (DMDD) because the latter is more extreme. Grossly out of proportion, severe temper tantrums occur at least three times a week for a year or more in two different settings (e.g., family, school) with persistently negative mood/irritability in between episodes. There isn't much research yet on disruptive mood dysregulation disorder, but its similarity to ODD means there may be shared risk factors. A child should not be diagnosed with both disorders, as the most severe takes precedence.[5]

WHAT IS IT LIKE TO PARENT A CHILD DIAGNOSED WITH ODD OR DMDD?

These are some of the most burdensome disorders regarding the daily grind, the negativity, and the emotional toll. Anything—and nothing at all—can lead to an argument. If you said the sky was blue, your child would say it was red, just for the sake of it. Kids with ODD and DMDD have a strong need to be "right" and "win." "No" is a trigger word, as is being told what to do. *Pervasive demand avoidance* is a term recently popularized in the autism parenting arena, but kids with oppositional/ defiant symptoms also will overreact and explode over the simplest of asks. Suppose you're a parent of a child with an oppositional, defiant, and angry/irritable disorder. In that case, you know the amount of time spent finessing events and activities to bring them off successfully. You may resent how much work and effort seem to go into the simplest, ordinary, and routine matters. As a result, some parents complain about the joy being sapped from family life because of the amount of planning required.[6]

Another stressor with raising these children is the public embarrassment. A child might act out in public in socially unacceptable ways (crying, yelling, screaming, hitting); people are watching and it feels like judging: what's wrong with that child? Why can't the parents control their child? All children have oppositional and defiant moments, but parents of children who do not suffer from ODD or DMDD will not understand the burden.

WHY IS MY CHILD LIKE THIS?

Like with many of the disorders discussed in this book, the current understanding is that genetic risk and environmental adversity are involved, perhaps with each contributing 50 percent.[7]

Biological

As newborns, children with a biological predisposition to these disorders may show a difficult temperament: they cry constantly, are difficult to soothe, and are irritable.[8] Families with kids diagnosed with ODD/DMDD often have a history of mental disorders, substance use disorders, and criminal offending.[9] There's an interesting relationship between depression in mothers and child ODD.[10] Risk for depression may already exist in mothers before the birth of their child, and parenting a child can feel defeating and demoralizing to most parents, much less those who already have a susceptibility to depression. Parents suffering from depression can be inconsistent about discipline, depending on their active symptoms (e.g., hopelessness, irritability, vegetative symptoms) and may have a negative bias. They may not have the energy for the extreme demands of caregiving that these kids require. Therefore, it is essential that if you suffer from depression or other mental health issues, you receive treatment for yourself (therapy and/or medication). See chapter 10 for more guidance.

Psychological

A typical psychological profile of kids with ODD and CD is impulsivity, low verbal intelligence, and social processing issues, which translates into a lack of social skills and self-control. Some of the deficits in social processing involve:

- Rigidity and inability to come up with solutions to a problem

- Difficulty identifying consequences of a choice and its effects on others
- Failure to grasp how others feel and their perspectives
- Attributing hostile motivations to the actions of others

When these kids feel wounded, even if it's only an accidental bump in the school hallway, they feel justified in lashing out and retaliating at a degree out of proportion to the original offense. For example, Sean reacted angrily to the coach laughing when he and other kids entered the gym. He swore at the coach, who then dismissed Sean from practice. As Sean ran out of the gym, he grabbed some paint that happened to be lying in the hallway and drew vulgar pictures in the snow. The escalation seemed to ignite when Sean reacted to his coach's laughing, obviously seeing ill intent. Fortunately, some recent intervention research showed that hostile attributions can be altered in DMDD with accompanying changes in the brain.[11]

Social

Peers

So-called normal children may fear and avoid an explosive child because of the negativity, argumentativeness, and explosiveness. Some kids with oppositional defiant features like to dominate others. In younger grades and middle school especially, they may be popular because they act in ways other kids find shocking or funny. Many of these kids will also have ADHD (ADHD and ODD are a prevalent combination), meaning they have difficulty inhibiting impulses. Kids of this type often consort together, egging each other on to more extreme behaviors.

Family

Protective factors are secure attachment, which is cultivated by sensitive, attuned, and empathic caregiving,[12] and positive, warm, and supportive parenting. However, it's difficult to feel warm when a child is bucking every request and being shockingly rude. Not to anyone's surprise, harsh parenting and psychological and physical abuse are risk factors.[13]

Conflict between parents is another risk factor.[14] Frequent arguing between parents models this behavior and creates a potentially volatile environment. Couples are at risk to separate and divorce partly due to child-rearing stressors. Single-parent status may worsen kid behaviors because there aren't two parents to bear the brunt of caregiving and discipline, the demands of which are formidable.

WHAT *CAN* YOU DO?

Self-Care

First, care for yourself, as raising a child who demands so much can feel defeating. Please do what you need to get time for yourself and participate in daily enjoyable activities, whether coffee, workouts, walks, arts, crafts, gardening, movies, seeing friends for meals, whatever it is for you. Of course, this is more difficult when children are young and you can't leave them alone, but when they're older, you have more latitude to make sure you take time-outs and leave the house to replenish yourself.

Support

The stress of parenting children with disruptive behaviors is more than most people can handle alone. Have a support system in place to help you make it through. Ask your partner to be on the same page and approach parenting with a unified front. If you have extended family members, lean on them for extra help. Being around your child can help family members understand the challenges you have. David's uncle spent 30 minutes trying to teach David's eight-year-old son how to fish but was exhausted by his inability to listen and impatience. He understood in a way that he previously could not when David simply related the daily challenges to him. Of course, what also may happen is that they behave for a short while with other people. The effort of "holding it together" might mean they release all the tension onto you. Once again, your parenting is doubted.

Friends can also provide support, though other parents may not understand your troubles because they haven't had similar experiences with their children. If you don't have anyone in your immediate circle, look outside for more formalized support. (See Resources and chapter 10.)

Try Not to Take Things Personally

Some parents recognize when their child is stuck in the grip of negativity, but others take hurtful comments personally: "Why is my child being so mean after all I do?" "Why does my kid hate me?" Trice likened her third-grade son to an abusive partner, which she'd never had because she wouldn't put up with that. She described her son's tirades: "I hate you. You're old, you're ugly, you're fat, you're a 'ho."

Kids diagnosed with ODD know how to "push your buttons" to get a reaction, which gives them a big charge. In behavioral theory terms, they receive reinforcement for this behavior. They seek out shock and outrage, even tears, and they relish in them. They become heady with their power and, drunk on it, become out of control.

It's easy to personalize because of the closeness of the parent-child relationship. But that very closeness provides the safety net for the child. They know they can count on you to love them unconditionally, and so will take frustrations out on you. Ultimately, it's not about how you *feel*; it's more important that you *respond* in a matter-of-fact and unemotional way toward their provocations.

Resist the Urge to Argue

Parents of kids diagnosed with these disorders must become adept at preventing, sidestepping, and disengaging from the child's almost constant invitations to fight. It takes a lot of self-control to squelch the natural reaction to jump in and become part of the argument, especially when your child refuses to do something. One major challenge in ignoring provocation and annoying behavior is identifying which behaviors warrant ignoring. The general guideline is that it's for bothersome but not unsafe behavior. It gets complicated when it comes to disrespectful or vulgar language. Most parents would want to leap into the fray and stop such behavior immediately, afraid that they were being permissive and "allowing" children to say awful things. The vulgar language and the disrespect can be handled in the moment like whining: "When you're ready to speak appropriately to me, then I'll talk to you." After, when everyone calms down, that is the time to address disrespect/language. As a starter, you might say, "When I was asking you to put your dishes in the dishwasher, you seemed to be having a lot of trouble. What was going on?"

One issue with ignoring explosions is that your child might feel abandoned when you pull away and don't say anything. They will interpret your lack of response as a form of rejection. As twisted as it seems, arguing with someone *is* a way to connect. When overwhelmed with vulnerability, children may express their feelings through rage and become even more aggressive. Trice would tell her son, "If you're going to talk to me like that, I'm not going to let you sit on my lap. When you can be respectful—even if you're angry—I'll talk." He'd cling to her and state, "You have to stay here and accept it because you deserve it." This is not to discourage you from setting a boundary but to prepare you for what may happen (and to validate you if it's already happened).

Conjure Up Empathy

It's not easy to empathize with kids who have challenging behaviors. I must remind myself that someone looking to cause pain is likely also feeling miserable. It seems these kids want to make everyone else just as unhappy as they are. So, if you feel annoyed, frustrated, and deflated, you can understand *their* feelings in that moment.

Children diagnosed with ODD/DMDD struggle to see things from another person's point of view. To enable them to experience empathy for other people, they must experience empathy. When Trice's son was without anyone to hang out with after school and began to act up, she tried to look past his behavior and said: "I can tell you're disappointed Rex isn't here today; you enjoy spending time with him so much."

Even then, some kids diagnosed with ODD might put up resistance. Teenage Rob tells his mother that she is speaking to him "like a dog" when she tries to show him empathy, so instead of using "feeling" words, she tries to be more subtle, using terms like *bummer* or *suck* that he deems more appropriate.

In *Love and Logic*, the authors Foster Cline and Jim Fay suggest leading with empathy if a child suffers a natural consequence.[15] For example, if a teen gets a ticket because of speeding, a scolding stance is to say, "I told you not to speed. You're going to have to pay for that!" In *Love and Logic*, you make more of a show of empathy: "I'm sorry you got a ticket. That's such a bummer to pay." Another typical example involves low grades: "That must feel so disappointing to get that grade. That's not what you were wanting." Contrast this with a typical statement, "See, I told you to study more. When are you going to learn?" If we harangue our kids, they fight against *us* and feel resentful rather than sitting with their lesson (e.g., if I speed, I might have to pay a ticket). The more you tell a child what they did was wrong, the less responsible they will feel.

Work with Child Strengths

Most parents naturally focus on their children's unique qualities and talents, like their quirky personality, compassion, flair for performing, or passion for animals. It's much easier to bolster what is already working for your child than to change behavior. Taylor noticed that while school, in general, and math, in particular, was challenging for her daughter, she had a natural empathy for animals, much more than she did for people. Therefore, Taylor joined an animal rescue organization to foster the occasional litter of puppies. It was a lot of work and responsibility, but her daughter was motivated like she hadn't been for anything else Taylor had tried, and mother and daughter could bond over this endeavor. Jackson was outgoing, coordinated, and good at team sports involving balls, so his mother kept him in two sports a season to structure his time, give him outside activity, and meet his social needs.

Avoid Physical Force

It's tough to manage an angry and explosive child, requiring vast reserves of patience. If you're around an older generation, like your parents, they may insist on the usefulness of physical punishment for aggressive and defiant behaviors. When so many things don't seem to work with your child, you may start to wonder, *Maybe some children need physical discipline. Maybe that is the only way to get through to my child.*

Physical force won't help either, though. Although your child might temporarily comply, it will be short-lived and won't generalize to the future. Violence and threats of violence beget more anger and aggression. Your child might take their behavior up to even more extreme heights and only obey at that point, which means you've trained them to disobey until you escalate to that level. You also might damage the relationship, cause trauma, and get in trouble legally yourself. It's not a good option, even when it feels like you're out of options.

Of course, at times, the best of parents become overwhelmed. Our anger, impatience, and frustration burst through, and we might become violent. If this happens, the best you can do is apologize: "I am sorry for hitting you yesterday. I became too frustrated and overwhelmed myself. What you did still wasn't right, and it's not okay to hit. I'm sorry. Next time, I'll leave the house until I feel calmer and can deal with the situation."

If your child threatens you with calling child protective services (CPS), tell them, "Do what you need to do." I know some parents have felt over a barrel when their children make these threats, but try not to overreact and certainly don't cave in. First, your child is probably only making threats. Second, even if your child does make a report, CPS personnel determine which calls to pursue and may not even bother with it. Only 55 percent of cases go on to have an investigation.[16] Third, if a CPS worker calls or comes by, tell them about the challenges you're having with your child and the services you're already pursuing. Ask if they can help with referrals or resources. Almost two million families received prevention services in the United States in 2021 after an investigation without CPS becoming involved in further monitoring.[17] In most investigations, CPS will not remove a child or become involved legally.

Change the Yelling Habit

Some parents admit to being "yellers" as it helps them release tension and frustration. Understand that yelling falls within the camp of "punishment," though. Consider that you may have inadvertently trained your child to disobey until you start screaming. If you yell a lot, this behavior is then modeled for your children, and they may escalate. They also tend to tune out your yelling, and it doesn't lead to more compliance. Yelling can become a habit, but, like any habit, can be changed.

Minimize Lecturing

Most parents lecture too much. We desperately want to convince our child of the "right" position, and we think telling them repeatedly and at length will translate into more understanding on their part. We want to teach and help our children and get things done, so we rush to answers and fix the problem.

When I led family sessions for parents with children with behavior problems, a beginning question was: "When therapy is successful, what will you see your child doing?" After parents spoke at length in answer, I would turn to the child and ask, "What did your mom just say?" The child could not answer most of the time, having tuned out and lost track many sentences ago. At that point, I would have the parent answer the question again briefly so their children could grasp the gist of the message and repeat it back. As a result of seeing this so many times, I try not to fall into the same trap, but my husband still has to gesture at times that I should just stop, so I understand how you desperately want to convince your child to behave.

However, lecturing is another punishment-based technique, and, as you know, it's more optimal and effective to rely on reinforcing and rewarding desired behavior rather than punishing misbehavior. As parents, we believe that the more we talk, the better our children will understand what we say. But the opposite, in fact, is true. The more we talk, the more they will tune us out.

Since it's hard to focus on what *not* to do, a replacement behavior is to ask questions, which will help them consider various aspects of the situation, put more responsibility onto the child, and get them more involved in problem-solving. If you can help it, avoid sarcasm and interrogations and lead with open-ended questions:

What happened?
What did you think was going to happen?
At any point, did you wonder whether this was a good idea?
What was your thinking then?
What do you think should happen now?
What ideas do you have for how to approach this?

Pick Your Battles

If you fought every battle with your child, you would be more exhausted than you already are, creating even more negativity in the household. You have to let go of some things and allow natural consequences. For example, if a child destroys something in their room, like a lamp, they either have to put up with overhead lighting or pay for a new lamp out of their allowance.

Or, as described by Dr. Robert Greene in the Lives in the Balance program, a more radical solution is letting go of certain expectations. Gillian's preschool son had daily tantrums and resistance around putting on socks and shoes. Therefore, she dropped the expectation that he would wear shoes. A couple of times in the playground, he minced around on the playground tan bark in 40-degree weather. Other mothers were appalled, but Gillian allowed it, armed with the science that being cold doesn't make you more susceptible to catching a cold. He finally landed on his sister's pink Crocs that he found tolerable as long as he didn't have to wear socks. Therefore, Gillian settled on his wearing those, finally solving the problem.

Handling Tantrums

Tantrums might look different, depending on the child's age: toddlers scream and throw themselves on the floor; school-age children throw things and slam doors; and teenagers punch holes and damage property. Many parents of children diagnosed with disruptive dysregulation mood disorder speak favorably of Dr. Matthews's protocol. Dr. Daniel Matthews, now retired, developed the protocol after running an inpatient program at Duke University for aggressive children. He likened tantrums to epileptic fits, not within the child's control. He was also surprised that children would remember very little about the tantrum afterward.

His advice for managing tantrums is to allow them to run their course. That means remaining quiet, taking other family members with you out of the room, and taking pains not to inflame it. He advises not to punish tantrums or even threaten consequences, as they involve a lack of voluntary control.

When children act in these ways, parents get dysregulated, too, with the volume, the volatility, and the negativity, which invokes helplessness, frustration, sadness, and heartbreak. Even if you manage these heavy reactions and do "the right thing," it will still not feel good.

Some parents try to hold their children during these episodes. (Others are so mad, that's the last thing they feel like doing.) Most children will reject physical touch, even as they secretly wish you could make them feel better. They try to punish you with how they feel. I would put it out there to your child that you're available for hugs and holding, if you are comfortable with that, when they're ready.

Some Discipline Tips

At times, there must be consequences, but, as I'm sure you've heard, try to make sure, when possible, that they are natural consequences. An explosive child will lose things, destroy possessions, and punch holes in walls. If they destroy something, then they should not get it replaced, and this goes double for expensive electronic devices. If they deface something, they must rectify or pay for the damage. If they lose something, they have to feel the pain of that loss and have to earn money/ give over allowance to pay for a replacement rather than your just telling them it's wrong.

Another tip from the Love and Logic program is that discipline doesn't have to be applied at that very moment. Many of us want to "fix" a situation or feel some control over it. We also wonder if it will impact our child more if it's delivered immediately. But if you wait, you are calmer, more reasoned, and will have had the chance to perhaps check in with the other parent or get some advice. For the child, the delay means that they (not you) must sit with the uncertainty of what will happen.

Triggers

As you probably already know, prevention is likely the best way to handle the triggers that set off your child, such as being tired, hungry, bored, or overwhelmed with a new or different circumstance. At times, that means not doing an event or activity that you might have expected pre-child to be a routine part of family life, such as errands, family getaways, and religious attendance.

You may have found that *no* is a trigger word. I was proud of my ability to say no since it seemed difficult for so many parents, and, in all fairness, that's what parent training advises. However, now I see it as unnecessarily escalating. That doesn't mean giving in. It means just getting rid of the word *no* with some of the following suggestions:

1. *Use imagination for wish fulfillment.* Dr. Laura Markham, who developed Aha Parenting, says that allowing children to experience the wish in their imagination has important benefits in itself.[18] "That would be a lot of fun to shop for your birthday now."

2. *Discuss your adult concerns in a way they can understand* (from Dr. Robert Greene from *The Explosive Child*): "Unfortunately, we have to drop by the grocery store to pick up food for dinner, and if I don't get it now, we won't have anything thawed that I can cook." "I'm concerned that if you eat candy before bed, your teeth will get cavities. It means you'll have to go to the dentist even more to get them fixed, you'll have to get a painful injection to numb your mouth, and it will be very expensive."

3. *Figure out how they can get their wish, perhaps offering choices*: "I'm not sure we'll have the time to do that. But we can do it tomorrow or would you prefer on Saturday?" Choices, in general, are better than a defiance-provoking "no": "You're welcome to get in the car dressed or to bring your clothes with you when I leave in five minutes."

Promote the Couple Relationship

If you're in a relationship, ensure it's stable and free of conflict and demonstrate polite, respectful, and assertive communication rather than arguing and irritability. Model how people express their feelings in safe and healthy ways, even when they disagree, and show that ruptures can be repaired. Couples counseling can help you better support each other in the stress of having a child with special needs (see chapter 10).

One major area for potential conflict is that parents come from two completely different perspectives on how to handle a child who is angry, explosive, and disrespectful. The explosive child will often home in on these differences and work them to personal advantage. A team approach is therefore necessary.

Inevitably, people get together as a couple because they complement each other, which means they come with two different perspectives and approaches. Some common styles are to have one person withdrawn and the other overprotective; another is coercive, the other parent is permissive. Compared to what it takes to parent a "typical" child, parents must come together in a way that takes far more skill, finesse, and patience.

It's also not fair when one parent is the disciplinarian (the "bad guy") and the other plays the "good guy" or "soft touch." Obviously, no one wants to create this setup; partners are ideally united in their parenting, supporting each other in that role. Both parents should be involved in parenting explosive children, even if one parent works and the other is stay-at-home. The main caregiver needs support, respite, and replenishment. Additionally, the parent who's often out of the home doesn't have a complete picture of what it's like to parent the child. I've seen many cases where the homemaker struggles daily with out-of-control child behaviors that might be eased with medication for the child, and the parent who doesn't do much in the way of caregiving takes a strong stance against it. Both partners need to work together to meet the challenges of parenting a child diagnosed with ODD/DMDD.

PARENT TRAINING

There is a large collection of evidence, going back from the current day to the last several decades, to support behavioral therapy, also called *parent training* and *behavioral management*. Hundreds of studies show that both parents and neutral observers rate children's behavior as improved compared to no treatment in a relatively short-term treatment period (twelve to sixteen sessions) and maintained over time.[19] Parental stress, maternal depression, and parenting skills also improve with behavioral therapy. There is much less research on the use of parent training with specifically DMDD, but that is because of the newness of the disorder. In a pilot study, parent training was found effective for aggression and behavioral problems, but not the irritability found with DMDD.

Behavioral parent training relies heavily on operant conditioning, or the concept that behavior is more likely to happen if it has been reinforced. Instead of reinforcing undesirable behavior, parents shift their attention to what they desire. Behavioral theory views parent and child interactions as escalating in a coercive cycle. Carol came to my practice with her nine-year-old son Will, who was diagnosed with ODD and ADHD. She described a pattern of engagement between them which started with a request: "Please do your homework." Will responded coercively with noncompliance—whining, yelling, crying. In turn, Mom either removed the *aversive stimulus* and dropped the request, or she raised her voice and posed threats to encourage compliance. Following that, Will often responded in two ways: compliance, thereby reinforcing the parent's aversive behavior; or, more often, escalation, which reinforced Mom's withdrawal of commands. In these interaction sequences, parent and child train each other to become increasingly aversive.

Reinforcement

Parents can use a variety of ways to reinforce their children's behavior:

- *praise* and other social reinforcers: hugs, pats on the head/shoulder, an arm around the child, a smile, a wink, a thumbs-up sign
- *high-probability behaviors*: behaviors the child is already doing, such as gaming, TV, other screen time, become dependent on the child meeting an expectation, such as chores or homework: "For six homework problems, you can have a half hour of phone time."
- *token economies*: tangible reinforcers, such as chips, coins, tickets, stars, points, stickers, or check marks, for desirable behaviors that are then traded in for an agreed-upon reward.

The advantages of token economies are many:

- They can initially procure high levels of performance from children.
- They bridge the gap between the desired behavior and the reward.
- Points can be attached to different tasks that may comprise a desired goal when the behavior involved is complex. For instance, "getting to school on time" comprises several behavioral sequences; therefore, each sequence can be reinforced rather than

waiting until the whole behavior is performed. In this way, behavior is shaped to a desired goal.
- Tokens can be quickly and easily administered without interrupting the desired behavior.
- Tokens are less prone to satiation. When rewards chosen lose their reinforcing value, they can be exchanged for other rewards.[20]

Although token economies can be very effective, one major drawback is that parents have to be organized about implementing them consistently. The following tips may help:

1. Keep the number of target behaviors to a minimum, possibly even just one.
2. Have modest goals to start, and don't make the math too complicated. Consider how much of a behavior, such as chores, the child is already doing. What is a reasonable goal (how many points) to earn a reward?
3. If multiple children live in the household, pick the same behavior for everyone.
4. Have children decorate the chart so they have buy-in.
5. Place the chart in a physical position where children can see.
6. Allow children to place stars or stickers themselves under your supervision.
7. Don't make the math too complicated to earn a reward.
8. Rewards need not cost money, and offering time with you on a game or something they want to do might be a great reinforcer.
9. Tailor rewards to the particular child to boost motivation.
10. 10. As children's behaviors take hold, you can require more of the same or a different behavior over time.

Ignoring

The definition of *ignoring* (also called *extinction*) involves no longer reinforcing a behavior, resulting in a decrease in the behavior or its possible eradication.[21] Carol negatively reinforced Will's begging and whining because he was allowed to get out of homework. Therefore, ignoring his behavior will break this connection (begging and whining = getting out of doing a demanding task).

Many parents with children diagnosed with ODD/DMDD complain that their children will follow them out of the room when they try to ignore the behavior. My suggestion is to start doing housework or yard work. First, you're already upset and frustrated; since you're unhappy, you might as well tackle something that's not fun. But the second reason is that you can then say to your child, "Okay, if you want to be with me, we can work together on this." In my experience, they will usually leave you alone at this point.

I prime parents that the process of breaking a previous pattern is gradual. Don't expect your child to give up immediately or after the first time. They will keep trying for a while because it has worked so well. There is also an *extinction burst*, in which, trying to get the reinforcement they are used to, the child will redouble their efforts to obtain it. Their behavior might become highly obnoxious to the point where they might tantrum. Hearing your child scream and cry might feel intolerable, but take it as a sign that your actions are working. If the child moves toward positive behavior, praise, no matter how negatively you feel.

For young children, ignoring should be accompanied by distraction. For instance, if a four-year-old cries because she wants to destroy the remote control, rather than shouting at her, Dad could take the remote control away and divert her attention to a brightly colored ball: "Here's something else you can play with. See if you can catch it!"

Setting Up Stimulus Conditions

Aside from reinforcement, you can set up a situation for success by preparing in advance. Children can enjoy drawing pictures of each stage of their morning routine: getting dressed, eating breakfast, brushing teeth, and so forth, and feel a sense of ownership rather than a routine imposed upon them. If you hang the pictures on the wall, everyone can track the sequence in the morning, and you can use them as prompts, for example, pointing at particular pictures and asking, "What do we need to do next?"

Modeling respectful interactions means making short, polite statements about what you want ("Please take your dishes to the sink") rather than what you don't want ("stop making a mess around here"). Sometimes, it's helpful to add your underlying adult concern à la *Lives in the Balance* because the child with the ODD/DMDD profile is so explosive regarding requests. They see ill-intent where there is none and feel "picked on" when you make a request. They appreciate it more when you pose it as necessary for work *you* have to do: "I need to be able to wash these dishes that are piling up in the sink, so first the dishwasher has to be emptied." In this example, I managed to avoid using *you* to take away any triggering accusatory language. Allow transition time rather than asking for task completion at that moment: "After this program is over, I'll need help with the dishes." "Get to a place in your game where you can finish up soon." Transitions can be challenging for these kids, with their tendency toward rigidity.

Consequences

Time-out from reinforcement is the suggested punishment (consequence) in this model in which the child is placed in a non-stimulating spot for a prescribed time, usually a minute for each year of age. Other consequences involve taking away privileges or doing chores. One of the fundamental guidelines is that a program needs to focus on reinforcement over punishments.

Programs

There are several empirically supported parent training programs, including Incredible Years (https://www.incredibleyears.com), Triple P (https://www.triplep.net/glo-en/home/), Parent Management Training (https://www.parentmanagementtraininginstitute.com), and Parent Child Interaction Training. As well as using behavioral therapy, parent-child interaction training focuses on the parent-child attachment with the idea that behavioral techniques will work better when there is a strong relationship. Part of the treatment involves the therapist coaching the parent supportively on how to interact with various child behaviors to reinforce desired ones. The American Academy of Pediatrics suggests that, at least for preschool children, families should participate in twelve weeks of parent-child interaction training. If your child is in preschool or early elementary school, qualified therapists can be found on the website: https://www.pcit.org/what-is-pcit.html.

Critiques

There's no debating the research evidence that backs up parent training,[22] but many parents have difficulty using it with kids with explosive and disruptive disorders. The impulsivity and short-term orientation might make it hard for these kids to be motivated by future reinforcement. Additionally, they seem to get defeated easily; if they see a reward as too out of reach, they give up rather than being motivated to work toward it. I've also seen cases where a reinforcement system becomes yet another topic to debate and argue about. Additionally, parents sometimes complain about the focus of parent training on just child behaviors when they are more interested in the underlying reasons for behavior. There are also some controversies around the specific technique of time-out, which may devolve into a power struggle for kids diagnosed with disruptive disorders. They will not go to time-out, so you have to threaten or drag them.[23] In other words, sometimes, time-out will escalate an already challenging situation. Some children will feel abandoned and overwhelmed with their feelings in time-out and act out accordingly.

Alternative approaches that lack research support but that many parents find appealing include *Lives in the Balance*, *Aha Parenting*, *1-2-3 Magic*, and *Love and Logic*. These, among others, are described in chapter 10, as they may also be effective for other disorders covered in this book, including autism spectrum disorders, ADHD, anxiety, and OCD.

INDIVIDUAL CHILD THERAPY

Most treatments for children identified with ODD or DMDD are directed at parents not because they are to blame but because they have to set up environmental conditions and learn skilled ways of reacting. Generally, individual therapy is not as effective as parent-involved treatments for children's disruptive behaviors. First, due to cognitive development, children are less able to benefit from individual treatment when younger than eleven. Second, children with ODD and DMDD tend to blame others for their problems and aren't motivated to change.

The most well-known individual therapy studied is Coping Power, developed to respond to social processing deficits: https://www.copingpower.com. Instead of reacting with aggression, the child learns how to interpret social situations accurately, figure out options, choose one that maximizes advantages, and practices the skills in role-play.[24]

SCHOOL

Many children with ODD and DMDD will also be diagnosed with ADHD. Chapter 1 covered the laws and interventions that the school can offer, including 504 accommodation and Individualized Education Plans (IEPs). Typically, kids diagnosed with disruptive disorders qualify for an IEP under the classification of "emotional disability." Services for an emotional disability may include regular counseling in the school, and, starting in middle school, an "instructional studies" elective, where the child gets a study hall period. Here they can receive help for assignments as needed. Schools will provide the "least restrictive setting" and center academic performance as an indicator of whether the child should remain in the mainstream classroom with supports or move to a specialized class or other placement.

Parents of kids with ODD and DMDD are often summoned to collect their children early because of unruly or out-of-control behavior. Make sure that you request that a signed letter from the principal documenting the suspension is ready when you arrive. School administration realizes that such documentation may build a case that your child requires more services, which by law, a public school has to provide.

If the services provided by the school don't seem to be making a dent and your child isn't improving at least slightly, my advice is to try to get the accommodations/placements to move faster. You can also call an IEP meeting yourself if you believe there is no progression; otherwise, the school administration takes a "wait and see" approach, which can involve a large proportion of your child's school year. Some parents hire an educational advocate familiar with the laws around special education to ensure that kids are getting their needs met in the school system. See chapter 9 and the Resources section, which supplies a website that provides questions to ask before hiring an education advocate.

However, and despite this advice, when you are with your child, it's important to take the school's side rather than your child's. A child with ODD or DMDD already has issues with authority (i.e., defiance), so we want to bolster the authority of the school and maintain a team approach. Meanwhile, you may be advocating behind the scenes for more effective services.

MEDICATION

Generally, experts suggest psychotherapy for aggressive behavior rather than solely medicating. That being said, medication is often needed due to out-of-control behaviors that impact essential domains of child, family, and school functioning. Due to the overlap with attention-deficit hyperactivity disorder (ADHD), the stimulants are prescribed for both oppositional defiant disorder (ODD) and disruptive mood dysregulation disorder (DMDD). Stimulants reduce aggression, possibly by controlling impulsivity.[25, 26]

Another drug used for aggression is the antipsychotic risperidone. Clinical trials spanning six and twelve weeks found a reduction in conduct problems and aggression in youth who took risperidone compared to those who didn't receive any.[27] However, taking this medication can result in adverse side effects, namely rapid weight gain and its associated metabolic impairment. Other antipsychotics haven't received the required research attention and, therefore, aren't FDA-approved, but psychiatrists occasionally prescribe them.

A parenting community has centered around a medication approach for disruptive dysregulation mood disorder (see https://www.rdmdd.org) named "Matthews's protocol" after Dr. Daniel Matthews, who developed it at an inpatient unit for aggressive children at Duke University. The protocol involves the use of anticonvulsant medications commonly prescribed for epileptic fits, administered specifically to children who tend to become "out of it" and unreachable during a tantrum, with little memory of the event afterward. According to the protocol, the first-line choice is the anticonvulsant Trileptal, followed by Lamictal and Vimpat as other options. As part of the protocol, the medication amantadine, commonly used for Parkinson's disorder, is also prescribed. Even though these medications are prescribed "off-label," without FDA approval or randomized controlled trials to support their use, many parents have found them helpful in managing their child's condition.

SUMMARY

The parenting burden for children diagnosed with explosive disorders is high, and parents require a high need for self-care and support. Working with a child when they are younger may prevent more expensive intensive treatment down the line. This chapter has covered many early-age parenting programs that can equip you with the knowledge and skills to manage an out-of-control and explosive child. It has also discussed some crosscutting parenting strategies and approaches that I have found helpful for families from research and experience. If you can catch problems early enough and treat them effectively, you will have more success than when kids become teenagers and you don't have the same control over their environment.

Chapter 8

Adolescent Conduct and Substance Use Disorders

Conduct disorder (CD) and substance use disorders (SUD) are discussed together in this chapter due to the high rate of co-occurrence between them; the regular use of cannabis, cocaine, barbiturates, tranquilizers, hallucinogens, and inhalants among adolescents is linked to having conduct disorder.[1] Additionally, the disorders share overlapping risk factors and interventions.

CD is a pattern marked by aggression and/or antisocial behavior involving aggression; destruction of property; deceitfulness/theft; and serious violation of rules. CD is classified within the disruptive behavior disorders group, which includes ODD[2] (see chapter 7).

Children who are diagnosed with ODD progress to the more serious behaviors associated with CD about 50 percent of the time,[3] and most kids with CD also meet criteria for ODD. (They're not given both because in the *DSM*, the principle is that the more severe disorder is the one diagnosed.)

Substance use disorders are defined as recurrent and uncontrollable use despite harmful consequences. They involve at least two of the following symptoms: *impaired control* (taking larger amounts/over a longer period, persistent desire to cut down use but unsuccessful, a lot of time devoted to getting the substance, cravings); *social impairment due to use* (unable to meet major role obligations, persistent/recurrent interpersonal conflict, important social, occupational, or recreational activities are sacrificed); *risky use* (when it's physically hazardous or causes physical or psychological problems); and *pharmacological effects* (tolerance and withdrawal). The prevalence of lifetime substance use disorders among adolescents in 2018 was 26 percent for alcohol, 15 percent for cannabis, and 13 percent for tobacco. Methadone, oxycodone (OxyContin), and hydrocodone (Vicodin) are some of the most widely prescribed opioids, but the synthetic fentanyl is responsible for the majority of overdose deaths in adolescents. Between 2019 and 2020, overdose mortality increased by 94 percent for adolescents and from 2020 to 2021 by 20 percent.[4]

E-cigarettes have rapidly increased in popularity, becoming a predominant substance of misuse among US youths. According to the most recent results of the Centers for Disease Control Youth Risk Survey, almost a third of high school students have tried electronic vapor products and 7 percent used them frequently.[5] Although the age for purchasing nicotine products has increased to twenty-one in the United States, 8 percent of youth surveyed said they bought the product themselves from a store. The prevalence of cannabis vaping in the United States and Canada among adolescents has doubled from 2013 to 2020.[6]

WHY IS MY CHILD LIKE THIS?

Biological

Twin and adoption studies show that adolescent substance use is moderately heritable.[7] The neurotransmitter system in the brain associated with addiction is dopamine and its associated genes. Interestingly, genetic factors may play a greater role among boys than girls for whom environmental factors may be a stronger predictor.[8] Adoption is a risk factor for children, perhaps partly due to genetics and other biological risks, such as lack of adequate prenatal care. Understand though that these risks are malleable based on post-adoption support. Similar to ODD (see chapter 7), early risk influences for CD and SUD include, as well as male gender, irritable temperament, and lack of emotional regulation.[9] While some experimentation with substances is normative in adolescence, early use of substances is a risk factor for developing problem use[10] and conduct disorder.[11] When Nikita's thirteen-year-old son was caught taking alcohol from their supply, his parents gave it to a friend of theirs to hold and keep safe. In other words, you might not be able to keep alcohol in your house if you have a risky teen who is looking to take advantage.

Psychological

One factor that protects against the development of CD or SUD is not having another mental disorder. Childhood ADHD, ODD, CD, and depression (but not anxiety) increased the risk for development of a substance-use disorder and for relapse after treatment.[12, 13, 14] As discussed in chapter 3, depressive disorders need to be identified in youth and treated to prevent youth from habitual use of substances to manage emotional pain. Related to the importance of treating comorbid conditions to prevent and manage CD and SUD, some parents fear that if their children use stimulants to manage ADHD, they will get the idea that they should take substances for problems. The research supports the opposite. Treating child and adolescent ADHD with stimulant medicine (see chapter 1) seems to reduce the risk of future SUD.[15]

Other psychological risk factors linked to CD and SUD include impulsivity, rebelliousness, risk-taking, callous-unemotional traits with lack of empathy and emotional unresponsiveness, and shallow affect with an uncaring attitude. In the *Diagnostic Manual*, the diagnosis of CD contains a subtype labeled callous-unemotional since these traits are associated with worse outcomes.[1617]

Social

In addition to genetic contributors, environmental factors can influence the development of conduct and substance use disorders:

- Family, including parenting style, parental mental disorder, household composition (having a lot of children), and partner conflict
- Peer influence and LGBTQ status
- Neighborhood adversity and social disadvantage.

Family

Parenting style has been examined in relation to conduct and substance use disorders. In a study of 5,500 youth tracked over time, the researchers categorized parenting styles and their association with teen antisocial behavior. The researchers expected a *coercive* style, described as high family conflict and low positive family climate, to relate to antisocial behavior, but only 15 percent of families fit this profile. Child maltreatment, which can also be part of this style, is associated with teen aggression.[18]

The researchers were surprised to learn that *disengaged* and *permissive* styles were also associated with conduct problems. A disengaged style was most common at over 40 percent and was characterized as low connectedness among family members with a lack of involvement by parents. As a result, teens seek direction from other disengaged peers who turn to deviant activities, such as criminal acts and substance use. Over 10 percent of families were described as *permissive*, meaning that though there was warmth and a positive relationship between parents and children, effective discipline was lacking. While a positive connection with the child is a protective factor,[19, 20, 21] a lack of effective discipline or inconsistent discipline[22] is detrimental. Permissive parenting at age three is a risk factor for adolescent irritability,[23] and in another study of over ten thousand twins, parental permissiveness was the strongest predictor of adolescent behavioral problems.[24] The last parenting style identified was *high functioning*, found in a significant proportion of families (34 percent). This style is described as low family conflict and positive family climate, parental involvement with children, effective discipline, and positive engagement.[25] Obviously, this style can be difficult to strike—to have both the warmth and supportiveness and discipline.

Another family factor studied is parental mental disorder, particularly depression, and its relationship to adolescent conduct problems.[26, 27] It probably comes as no surprise that drug use dependence in parents is associated with substance use disorders in youth.[28] Similarly, lower marital satisfaction between parents when a child is a preschooler is associated with teen aggression and irritability, particularly for girls.[29] Being present during conflict is already stressful, but children also pick up on how to manage feelings and conflict from parents arguing and bickering. The implication is that if parents are struggling with mental health or relationship problems, there is no better advantage to provide than getting treatment for these issues. (See chapter 10 for discussion of how to access high-quality care for yourself and/or partner.) You may not only show up more consistently as a parent, but also model how to seek help and to manage stress and conflict better.

A final way family life influences development of CD and SUD is through household composition, namely increased family size (more than three). I worked at a justice system– involved community moni-toring program and would sometimes seek to motivate youth who were concerned about the impact of their behavior for their younger siblings, knowing that they were potentially modeling this kind of future for them. More children often means that resources—financial, physical, and emotional—are strapped. Also, monitoring and keeping up with multiple children is difficult.

Peers

Peers who use substances place an individual at risk, whereas friends who do not support such use are protective against the development of alcohol and drug problems. Consorting with non-substance-using peers after treatment also protects a youth against relapse.[30] Parents often talk about the "wrong crowd," and it can certainly be the case that deviant peer groups reinforce their members into more risk than they would alone.[31] However, it's more often "birds of a feather flock together," and a teen consorts with others like themselves.

You may have to take drastic measures to decrease your child's involvement with certain people for their own protection. There was recently a sad case in my area of a child who had started hanging around the "wrong crowd" in middle school. His parents fraudulently claimed an address in a better school system and got him out of the feeder high school in their area. However, their son still hung around his neighborhood group when he was not at school or with his sports teams. He unfortunately ended up dying in a drug-related robbery at eighteen before he'd graduated from high school with a committed college sports position. Reflecting on that case, I wonder if even more extreme measures were called for, such as the family selling their house and renting in a neighborhood in the new school district. I reflect on drastic measures because it's difficult, unless you operate at the neigh-borhood level, to break up potentially unsafe friendships. If children are in middle or high school, telling them not to hang around certain people only makes that group more enticing. As much as possible, work with child strengths, such as sports and interests, to steer children away from problematic influences.

In chapter 3, there was discussion of the risk for LGBTQ youth for depression. Similarly, LGBTQ youth are at particularly high risk for substance misuse, which results from the increased social stigma, discrimination, and psychosocial stressors.

Neighborhood

Neighborhoods can also provide risk or protection. A hallmark of ODD/CD is a bias toward seeing threat and hostility in others and then responding in a way that appears justified. However, youth living in impoverished environments may actually view adults involved in criminality, community violence, gangs, weapon-carrying, and aggression.[32] Exposure to these threats may naturally condition youth to view others as hostile and dangerous. Early social disadvantage might affect neural development, which may, in turn, influence behavior.[33, 34] Further, parents stressed by attending to basic needs may not have the energy and resources to devote to sensitive parenting. Children who grow up with social disadvantages may also have low aspirations for the future. Believing that the future is predetermined, they may see their actions and behaviors as having little to do with opportunities for adult success.[35]

Youth who have experienced exposure to traumas, including child maltreatment and other adverse childhood events, are more at risk for juvenile offending and criminal recidivism.[36, 37] Traumatic exposure may operate on delinquency through the mediating factors of coping by detachment and not caring.[38]

Availability of substances is associated with problematic substance use.[39] Parents might be worried about the impact of legalization of cannabis for teens. A review of US medical marijuana laws found they didn't increase the prevalence of adolescent marijuana use.[40] Neither was the proximity and density of medical marijuana dispensaries related to adolescents' current use or susceptibility to use marijuana.[41] Medical marijuana legislature was, in fact, associated with declines in use among male, Black, and Latinx adolescents, and decriminalization predicted significant declines in marijuana use among Latinx adolescents but significant increases among white adolescents.[42] While smoking of marijuana declined in adolescents following legalization, other modes of ingestion increased, such as edibles and dabbing.[43] The term dabbing is jargon that refers to the inhalation through a vaporizer of extremely concentrated tetrahydrocannabinol (THC) derived from marijuana-based oils, concentrates, and extracts.[44] The problem with this practice is that, in addition to concentrations of up to 80 percent compared to the 15–25 percent potency of smoking cannabis, home-made dabs and/or dabs from undependable sources may contain toxic substances including butane, pesticides, fungi, and bacteria, and have been linked to lung injuries secondary to the inhalation of concentrated cannabis. Because of the high concentration levels, dabbing may lead to increased susceptibility to addiction in developing brains. The common guideline is that cannabis usage be delayed until frontal lobe development is complete, which can be up to twenty-five years of age.

WHAT *CAN* YOU DO?

1. Teenagers with conduct and substance use issues should have a reasonable curfew to protect themselves, even though they will inevitably say that no one else has a curfew (that's not true). Allowing them to roam freely at night inevitably leads to trouble.
2. Cameras and alarms: Not everyone owns a home or has the resources so this may not apply, but security cameras and alarms have proven helpful for parents dealing with curfew violations or teens sneaking out. Cameras can also show you who comes to the house when you're not there.
3. Drug testing teens is a controversial practice, but if you choose to go this route,e here are some tips that might make it go more smoothly:
   a. Rather than surprising them, it's better to let your child know in advance that drug testing will happen. Then when you produce a drug test, have them do it immediately by drinking water until they can provide a sample without them being able to go to their rooms or anywhere else.
   b. Online stores offer affordable drug tests, or you can ask your pediatrician or child's psychiatrist to order one. An order ensures that insurance will cover it; otherwise, they cost hundreds of dollars at a lab service.
   c. If there is any resistance or delay when you present a drug test, consider it a failed test to avoid being strung along.
   d. Note there are also tests available for nicotine due to the rise of vaping. These tests can help ensure your child stays clean from

nicotine. Make phone privileges contingent on that since the phone may be used in some manner to obtain vaping supplies.

e. Clean drug tests are required to earn privileges, particularly driving, curfew, and screen time.

f. Steel yourself for a potentially negative, defensive interaction when you request a drug test, although strive for a matter-of-fact tone.

g. Timing: Weekly or random but regularly enough that your teen is accountable.

INTERVENTION

Most adolescents (80 percent) receive SUD treatment on an outpatient basis,[45] although it may be intensive outpatient (three-to-five times a week). Other settings for youth with SUD and/or CD are inpatient hospitals, day treatment, residential placement, and, at times, incarceration. See chapter 10 for more details on some of these settings as they cross-cut disorders.

What Treatments Are Offered within Facilities?

The majority of treatment settings both for adults and adolescents use a twelve-step Alcoholics Anonymous (AA) or Narcotics Anonymous (NA) model. The AA stance is that alcohol is a progressive disease and that, due to underlying vulnerabilities, certain people, called "alcoholics," can only strive for total abstinence. Because of the lure of alcohol, only a higher power, defined by each individual, even if it's only the power of the group, can help restore people to sanity. AA approaches are also called "twelve-step" as there are a series of steps in which members work with a sponsor, a person who has achieved a significant amount of time in sobriety. Although teens may learn about the philosophy of AA and attend twelve-step meetings as a part of their treatment, follow-up after treatment tends to be low for teens. A quarter of teens when surveyed say they don't relate to any aspect of AA. Meetings will also tend to be populated by adults, and abstinence as a goal might not resonate with teens.[46] Al-Anon attendance for you and other family members might be helpful for coping and support if your teen has an ongoing addiction.

Evidence-Based Treatment

Cognitive-Behavioral Therapy

Cognitive-behavioral therapy is a "well-established" treatment for adolescent substance use disorders. It's often delivered in a brief time frame (five to twelve sessions) and either in group or individual formats. The core elements include the following:[47]

Functional analysis of behavior problems involves identifying the typical scenarios in which substance misuse occurs and its triggers and analyzing the reasons for use and their disadvantages.

Prosocial activity sampling: restructuring everyday environments to avoid high-risk persons and situations and seek new outlets for social and recreational activities.

Cognitive monitoring and restructuring: gaining awareness of how thoughts and core beliefs influence emotions and behaviors; learning to view events or behaviors in a new light; and using reason, and/or considering alternatives.

Emotion regulation training: anger management and relaxation training.

Problem-solving training: Identifying stressors, breaking them down into manageable problems, brainstorming solutions, analyzing and weighing the advantages and disadvantages, and selecting an option to use.

Communication training: active listening, negotiation skills.

Family Therapy

Family therapy models are suggested for adolescent substance use disorders, CD, and for youth involved with the juvenile justice system.[48, 49] The following models have been studied:

Family behavioral treatment: A thorough assessment is done to understand the factors that reinforce substance use and then the youth is taught strategies to avoid/manage triggers.[50] Parents are involved so they can supervise and monitor new routines and therapeutic homework and provide rewards to children for implementing strategies.

This treatment is relatively brief: sixteen to twenty sessions that range from one to two hours spread out over a one-year period. https://familybehaviorther.wixsite.com/familytherapy.

Treatment Foster Care Oregon (formerly Multidimensional Treatment Foster Care): In this model, youth are placed in a specially trained foster home for six to nine months and given intensive support and treatment involving a daily token reinforcement system. Individual weekly therapy sessions focus on problem-solving skills, anger expression, social skills development, and educational or vocational planning.[51] https://www.tfcoregon.com/

Functional family therapy.[52] Interactions between family members rather than the adolescent's behavior is the major focus. Techniques include changing beliefs, cognitions, expectations, and reactions between family members. FFT involves eight to twelve sessions for mild cases and up to thirty hours of direct service. https://www.fftllc.com/fft

Multidimensional family therapy is a multicomponent intervention targeting individual (communication skills, social competence, and abstinence-related skills), peer, school, and family risk factors.[53] MDFT can be delivered from one to three times per week over the course of three to six months depending on the treatment setting and the severity of adolescent problems and family functioning. https://www.mdft.org/

Multisystemic therapy.[54] Targets the different systems a troubled youth might be involved with: the individual child, parents, family, school, and peers. Families are seen two to three times a week in intensive services that last for about four to six months. https://www.mstservices.com/

School Interventions

Much of the information that was covered in chapter 1 on school involvement will be relevant here, since so many kids with CD, SUD, and other behavior challenges will have been diagnosed with ADHD. Most of the time, kids with antisocial features need an Individualized Education Plan, which is most often under the category of *emotional disability*. That way, if your child acts out in ways that gets them into trouble, such behaviors can be seen in light of previously established disabilities rather than as a disciplinary problem that deserves an in- or out-of-school suspension. Sometimes school administrators will suspend a child and claim that they don't have the resources to manage the behavior. However, legally, they do have to provide a free and accessible education, so there are other resources that can be used, such as putting the child into a contained classroom or finding and paying for a school setting that is set up to manage such behaviors.

I'll also mention again that requiring documentation (a signed letter from the principal) upon picking up your child for a suspension is a must. This will act to curb school official tendencies toward the overreaction that these kids often generate with their behaviors. School personnel are aware that documentation takes the decision into the legal realm, which is that a public school by law has to supply a free education based on the child's abilities. Repeated suspensions signal that the school may have to provide more resources so the child can succeed. Generally, school personnel will be cautious about setting that precedent.

Mobile Applications

An interesting study was just completed on a mobile app called iKinnect for conduct disorder in youth. Behavioral problems improved in a randomized controlled trial of iKinnect compared to a mobile tracking device (the control group). The authors believed that positive changes were due to more clarity around parental expectations and consistency in responding.[55] Because the control group also did well on some domains, it may be worthwhile getting a mobile tracking device for teens (the study used Life360). As of this writing, there is still an opportunity on the website to become a participant in a research study: https://www.ikinnectapp.com.

VIOLENCE AND JUVENILE JUSTICE INVOLVEMENT

A child with conduct disorder can become involved with the juvenile court for criminal activity, such as vandalism, car theft, or assault, and over 50 percent of youth detained meet criteria for conduct disorder.[56] If arrested, your child may be detained. Viola's son had brushes with the law: He'd been put in handcuffs for running around on a school rooftop; police called her to pick up her son for underage drinking; and he was a passenger when the driver lit a firecracker and threw it into another kid's car window. She and her husband had informed him that they would not hire a lawyer if he got into more serious trouble. He would be responsible as he'd already had near misses many times and should have learned from these.

Youth to Parent Violence

Child to parent violence is not commonly discussed, but it does occur within families, especially with children diagnosed with conduct disorder (aggression is part of the diagnostic criteria).[57] There are different reasons for child-to-parent violence. One involves modeling in that a parent might be in or was previously in a violent relationship, and the child witnessed the abuse. Often it's because the child wants something (or doesn't want to do something) and escalates to the point of being violent, or because they are becoming too wound up to manage their distress another way.

Parents who are recipients of their child's violence feel a sense of shame, stigma, and hopelessness.[58] Some mothers speak about feeling like they're living in an abusive relationship, which they can't leave because it involves their child. I've included a wonderful resource that was created by a local government in the UK about this topic: https://www.proceduresonline.com/nesubregion/files/southtyne_cpv.pdf. Although some of the specific resources they cite are UK based, a lot of the information they provide, including setting safety plans, are relevant to other audiences. Recall also chapter 7 and the advice for temper tantrums for older children, involving Matthews's protocol: disengage, leave the room, and take other children with you until the tantrum has expended itself.

If safety is an issue, call the police. The range of law enforcement response will vary, in part because of different jurisdictions, and also because individual police officers have a great deal of latitude in how they handle their cases. Some officers will say, "This is a family matter, not a criminal one" and leave. Some will try to talk to your child and warn them about potential consequences. Some will ask whether you want your child detained and will base their decision on that. Depending on the seriousness of the assault, a police officer might decide to bring charges. Being arrested equates to being detained, and your child might be removed and put in a detention center for a night.

Child in Need of Supervision

There are Child in Need of Supervision statutes for every state but most parents aren't familiar with them. They involve a petition that can be filed in the juvenile/family courts by various parties, including parents, that the child can no longer be safely contained in the home setting. A judge will order that the child and, possibly the parent, attend services, such as mandating the child for intensive outpatient substance use disorder treatment or in-home services. The county may pay for these services if money is an issue, which may be a huge advantage given the cost of treatment.

One major disadvantage is the child becoming embroiled in the justice system. Once a judge orders specific interventions, they have to be abided by. That means no more voluntary action; you'll have to do what's stated. Also, judges can be mercurial and ill-informed. For instance, they can mandate that your child goes to foster care. That might be okay if it's an evidence-based program like Treatment Foster Care Oregon, which is limited to nine months. More likely, it would involve garden-variety foster care, the quality of which ranges considerably for an unspecified length of time. You can't get your child and family out of the system quickly if you decide that it's no longer needed or you don't like the direction. Because it's a legal system, you then have legal responsibilities and mandates.

MEDICATION

The research on medications for adolescent substance use disorders is scarce and has tended to show no impact.[59] Many of the medicines used for conduct disorder and related problems are similar to the ones discussed in chapter 4. A review looked at the range of studies on medicines for antisocial problems and found many different types: the antipsychotics, atomoxetine, lithium, clonidine, divalproex sodium, and stimulants. Unfortunately, there is limited evidence regarding

pharmacotherapy's role in CD.[60] For one of the antipsychotics, risperidone, clinical trials found a reduction in both conduct problems and
aggression in youth who took it compared to those who didn't receive
treatment.[61] However, taking this medication can result in adverse side
effects, namely rapid weight gain and its associated metabolic impairments. Other antipsychotics that haven't received the required research
attention and, therefore, aren't FDA approved, are also occasionally
prescribed by psychiatrists.[62]

SUMMARY

This chapter discusses conduct disorder and substance use disorders, highlighting the overlap in risk factors and interventions. The
chapter suggests several strategies for parents to address teen conduct and substance use issues. Evidence-based treatments, such as
cognitive-behavioral therapy and family therapy, and school interventions are recommended. In more severe cases involving violence or
criminal behavior, involvement with the juvenile justice system may
be necessary. Overall, a comprehensive approach involving multiple
interventions and supports is essential in addressing adolescent conduct
disorder and substance use disorders.

PART V

Services

Chapter 9

Accessing Services and Navigating the System

This chapter delves into the realm of services, resources, and valuable tips for navigating mental health, social services, and criminal justice systems to obtain timely and high-quality assistance for your child and family. While previous chapters have explored these services, this chapter focuses on help-seeking across disorder, as many youth show more than one mental health challenge.

EARLY INTERVENTION

If preschoolers show significant behavioral issues and developmental delays, advocating for your child is crucial. As you may be aware, pediatricians have demanding schedules with brief patient appointments of no more than fifteen minutes. Furthermore, their training in mental health is generally limited to a basic level. Often, the parents, rather than the pediatricians, are more attuned to recognizing delays in their children's development. While it's true that pediatricians frequently encounter anxious parents whom they are accustomed to reassuring, not all concerns should be dismissed, as parents sometimes have valid worries.

Similarly, preschool teachers are becoming more proficient in identifying potential issues but may not always recognize underlying problems unless there are noticeable behavioral disruptions. Additionally, depending on the specific preschool and its staff, they may not be fully aware of community resources available. To overcome some of these limitations and barriers, you can contact your local public school district and request an evaluation. The Centers for Disease Control (CDC) offers a comprehensive, step-by-step process on how to access screening and assessment for your child before they enter school, which can be found at this link: https://www.cdc.gov/ncbddd/actearly/concerned .html. Having your child undergo an evaluation will provide you with valuable information about your child's abilities and needs, and it may qualify them for essential services. Research consistently demonstrates that early intervention is the most effective strategy for setting your child up for success.

SETTINGS

This section provides a brief overview of the different settings within the mental health system. Outpatient treatment (once a week for forty-five minutes) is usually the initial approach for children and adolescents. Only if this proves ineffective should more intensive intervention settings, such as intensive outpatient programs, partial hospitalization/ day treatment, psychiatric hospitalization, or residential treatment, be considered. Intensive outpatient treatment involves children attending therapy sessions at least three times a week. This approach may be suitable for various reasons, such as participation in a dialectical behavior therapy program that includes individual therapy, multifamily group sessions, and parental involvement. Some substance use and eating disorder treatment centers also employ intensive outpatient programs for adolescent clients.

Partial Hospitalization entails clients spending six to ten hours daily, three to seven days a week, in a hospital setting. These programs are often utilized as a "step down" after a child is discharged. However, they can also serve as an alternative to hospitalization if the risk is not severe. I have had self-harming clients who attended partial hospitalization programs without requiring a higher level of care.

Home Visiting is an intensive intervention where providers visit the child and family at home for a designated amount each week. The advantage of this approach is that it eliminates the need to organize transportation for short visits. Providers can observe and intervene in the child's natural environment. One potential disadvantage is that home-visiting providers often don't hold more than a bachelor's degree and have limited training and experience. Additionally, the designated time for home visiting may sometimes result in "filler time," where little progress occurs, and the provider simply spends time with the child. In theory, home visiting serves as a valuable method that bridges the intensity gap between outpatient therapy and placing the child in an out-of-home facility.

Hospitalization involves admitting the child to a medical or psychiatric unit in a hospital setting where multidisciplinary services are available. The point when hospitalization is considered is when your child is at risk of hurting themselves (self-harm, suicidal behaviors) or others (attacking, threatening to hurt/kill). Parents are heartbroken when they admit a child to the hospital. It's a difficult decision to make that your child is at risk of hurting themselves or others and that things have hit such a low point.

Another stressor is the difficulty of making these arrangements, depending on your location and your financial access to care; it's not an easy process to navigate, and you may have to leave multiple messages, be placed on hold, transferred, or on an unending waitlist. Accessing hospitalization for your child can be a complex process. Mental health providers often advise seeking emergency room care during a crisis, but this can be burdensome given long wait times in emergency departments. A social worker or other mental health professional at the hospital will evaluate your child's safety. Most of the time, the decision is that the child should go home with a follow-up plan to see a therapist and psychiatrist. To navigate this process, call your child's psychiatrist when things are at a crisis point, and the emergency line if they don't respond. This provider should assist you in making arrangements by calling the hospital. It's *not* advisable to show up at a local inpatient hospital with your child, as it can result in long wait times for screening or potential denial of service. If the inpatient hospital doesn't have beds available for new admission, they refer to other inpatient hospitals in the area, which may, unfortunately, be hours away from where you live.

During their stay, your child will room with other children and is monitored closely through frequent checks by the mental health aides, who deliver most of the direct care on the unit. Children twelve and under usually stay on one floor, and teens separated by gender are on another.

Understand that when a child is admitted, medication is a central part of the regime. Your child may be placed on more or different medications and perhaps an additional one by the time they leave the hospital. The other modality in this setting is group therapy. Nurses or mental health professionals offer different types of groups throughout the day. There may be one individual therapy session per week, and that person may also serve as the family therapist when your child is getting ready to leave. Usually, a child is hospitalized for a week.

Visiting hours for family members are generous, usually offered twice a day for an hour or two. Family members' packages and bags are searched, and they can't take cellphones or any other electronic devices into the unit. Many family members bring takeout food for their child, assuming that hospital food isn't the best and to offer a form of nurturance. Most kids plead with their parents to go home during visits and phone calls that generally take place in the evening. Parents find it heartrending to have separated their child from their home, albeit for extreme circumstances.

You may wonder what happens to their schooling if they're hospitalized. Contact the school after your child has been hospitalized and let your child's counselor know what has happened. School administration shows a lot of leeway and latitude for students who go through an experience like this. They don't want to put more pressure on the child. During an inpatient stay, a child will have a portion of the day devoted to academic work. You can pick up a packet of worksheets from the school that your child can do during this time.

The school will hold confidential that your child is in the hospital, and other kids will not know. After hospitalization, sometimes a child will be referred for one to three weeks at a partial hospitalization program. Again, some schoolwork will be completed each day, and the school will typically not expect your child to do homework at night.

Residential Treatment

Residential Treatment Centers (RTCs) provide a therapeutic environment outside of hospitals where clients reside for an extended period while receiving individual and group therapy. This type of setting becomes necessary when a child's behavior is severely disruptive to the point where they cannot function safely at home or school, affecting their well-being and that of others. RTCs cater to youth facing significant mental health challenges that have proven difficult to address in less restrictive settings.

RTCs grew out of their association with family courts. While youth without any arrests, offenses, or convictions cannot be detained in secure facilities, they can be mandated to receive treatment in RTCs.[1] RTCs serve youth from juvenile justice and child welfare systems, as well as those who have not been criminally charged. RTCs are divided into two distinct systems: those that are more expensive and privately funded in which parents and insurance companies pay for services; and government-funded programs that serve youth living in poverty. The private programs serve both male and female patients who are typically from wealthier families, while the government-funded ones mostly involve male patients from ethnic minority backgrounds who are involved in the juvenile justice or child welfare systems.

Wilderness Programs

Wilderness programs are in the category of residential treatment and are a group-intensive experience. Group sizes range from program to program but tend to be between six and ten clients. Therapeutic group gatherings, team building, and daily living conditions in the wilderness present challenges that require group cooperation and communication. Three types of wilderness therapy programs exist, depending on the length of intervention and the extent to which expedition backpacking or base camping is the primary mode:

1. Very short-term (a maximum sixty-day stay), continuous trekking expedition, which uses hiking, camping, and backpacking in groups on a wilderness route.
2. Short-term residential programs designed to last until the adolescent has made significant progress, typically ranging from six to twelve weeks. Participants live in groups at a base camp for most of the program and embark on ten- to fourteen-day wilderness backpacking treks.
3. Long-term residential programs consisting of participants living together in camps or groups in wilderness or rural settings

typically last nine to twenty-four months and incorporate wilderness aspects into everyday living.[2]

More studies have accumulated on wilderness programs than in the past. However, the research is still limited by lack of control conditions (kids that have similar issues but don't receive the wilderness intervention) and follow-up after youth leave these communities and return to live with their families.[3] In examining changes in youth from program entry to leaving, overall results were improvements in areas of self-concept, behavior changes, and clinical symptoms like depression.[4] Therefore, results are promising.

Educational Consultants

Parents often struggle to determine the appropriate destination for their children and want to ensure they choose a vetted facility. Educational consultancy has emerged as one of the businesses associated with the "troubled teen industry" as described by Dr. Frederic Reamer and Dr. Deborah Siegel. Educational consultants assist families in finding suitable placements and possibly tracking the child's progress during treatment. While educational consultants are privately paid, they adhere to a code of ethics through the Independent Educational Consultants Association that prohibits them from receiving "kickbacks" or special perks for recommending specific treatment centers or camps over others. Reamer and Siegel state that while the Independent Educational Consultants Association has done much to professionalize and advance the quality of its profession, such as requiring a master's degree, membership in IECA is voluntary.[5] Parents pay out of pocket to educational consultants.

Transportation Assistance

Transportation assistance is another service that parents pay for out of pocket to ensure that out-of-control and defiant children reach their treatment destination. Typically, the service, represented by a pair of burly adults, is scheduled in the early morning hours. The parents first enter the child's room and announce something like, "Scout, we love you, but I think you know things haven't been working out here for a while, so you're going to a place that can do more than we can to get you help."

From there, the pair from the transportation service drives the child to the placement or takes a flight. The purpose of this process is not only to ensure compliance but also to avoid any public or potentially unsafe incidents, such as a child attempting to run away during transportation. The colloquial term for this transportation service is "being gooned." It's important to note that wilderness programs are often considered an initial intervention to stabilize and prepare youth for further residential treatment settings.

Therapeutic Boarding Schools

Therapeutic boarding schools are residential schools that combine educational classes with group therapy, typically in a private, self-contained facility that runs year-round.[6] They are considered more voluntary than a residential treatment center and are not locked facilities. More information on therapeutic boarding schools and similar programs is available in the Resources section, although there is no national register or federal oversight.[7] Therapeutic boarding schools are paid for out of pocket by parents and can be, of this writing, around $100,000 a year.[8]

SCHOOL-BASED SERVICES

Children with mental health disorders often have either a 504 (see chapter 1) or an Individualized Education Plan, but not necessarily so. Generally, the school is more willing to become involved when symptoms result in failing grades, although there are widespread differences in how individual schools enact federal laws. This website gives parents much more information about how to obtain an IEP: https://www.understood.org/en/articles/evaluation-rights-what-you-need-to-know.

The process of an IEP is initiated by sending a formal letter addressed to the school. In this letter, kindly request that your child undergo an evaluation due to the adverse effects of their difficulties on academic performance. According to legal regulations, the school must arrange an interdisciplinary meeting involving key individuals, such as the principal or assistant principal, a school counselor, a social worker, a teacher, and parents. During this meeting, the aim is to determine whether there is enough justification to proceed collectively.

It's important to note that the specific actions taken by schools can vary significantly depending on the state and district policies. Some schools may only pursue additional measures if your child's grades have been significantly impacted. This issue may arise more frequently in schools where students are promoted despite their inadequate performance or in those where grade inflation has become prevalent, spanning all levels of education, including college and graduate school, in recent times.

What Kind of School Is Best for My Child?

Public schools possess greater resources for children with diverse needs and are bound by educational laws. Some parents may contemplate transferring their child from a public school to a more "traditional" private institution that offers smaller class sizes. However, unless catering to specific educational needs is their primary focus, private schools are ill-equipped to accommodate students with a wide range of abilities and requirements. Additionally, private education comes at a cost, which can be prohibitive and may not guarantee the best services. Another advantage of public schools, provided they are located in your area, is that they encompass children from your neighborhood. This allows your child to establish connections with local peers, fostering a stronger bond with the school. As part of their work, educational consultants determine the most appropriate school setting for your child.

Some parents hire educational advocates to help them navigate the special education system in their schools and advocate for increased or more specialized services. For instance, if your child cannot succeed in a mainstream classroom, they can be moved to a self-contained classroom with extra support. If that still proves difficult for your child, the school has to pay for more intensive services elsewhere in the district. There are no requirements for someone to call themselves an advocate, but many are from the education system or are lawyers. The Resources section has an interview guide if you're considering hiring an advocate.

Always request written documentation if your child is dismissed from school because of behavior. This documentation builds a case that current arrangements aren't serving the child, who may need a higher placement level. Aware of this fact, administrators will show more caution in suspending your child.

PROVIDERS

Primary Care Doctors

In any assessment for a mental disorder, a physical exam and labs are necessary to rule out any conditions that might mimic or explain symptoms. Pediatricians now routinely screen for depression and anxiety in annual visits, can make referrals for treatment, and often prescribe medicine. They also track weight and height trajectories.

Medical providers (nurses, doctors, nurse practitioners, and physicians' assistants) often discuss medication as a first-line option, given that their fields involve medicines. If your child responds to the doctor's prescribed treatment, then all is good. However, it can sometimes not be so easy to get a good response. At that point, pediatricians, rightly so, suggest a specialist in child psychiatry. Due to time constraints—sessions are often scheduled at fifteen-minute increments—and lack of training, primary care providers are sometimes ill-equipped to assess and manage a mental health disorder. Therefore, much variation exists among providers. They are also used to a dizzying array of parental concerns and almost reflexively dismiss them. The rampant reassurance is usually fine, but sometimes, getting an early diagnosis and services is a missed opportunity.

Psychiatrists

Psychiatrists are medical doctors who have an additional residence in psychiatric training. Currently, most psychiatrists only prescribe medication and do not undertake any psychotherapy. There is a severe lack of child psychiatrists in the United States, particularly in certain states and in rural areas. Because of the shortage, it may be difficult to find a psychiatrist who is taking new patients, depending on your area. In some major urban areas, like the DC metro where I live, most psychiatrists do not accept insurance and ask for the full fee at the time of service, which can run into the hundreds for an initial assessment and about $250 for a fifteen- to thirty-minute follow-up session. The benefits of psychiatrists are that they have received specialized training on mental disorders and their practice centers around prescribing medication for these conditions.

Other Psychiatric Providers

Because of the shortage of prescribers, other medical professionals, namely nurse practitioners and physicians' assistants with a psychiatric specialization, are supplementing the work of psychiatrists. Nurse practitioners have a doctoral degree and physicians' assistants have a master's degree with an additional specialization in psychiatric practice. These providers will likely assume more and more of the medication management for children with mental health diagnoses.

Psychologists

Doctoral-level psychologists (PhD) have been specifically trained in psychological testing. In a psychoeducational assessment, a psychologist performs a full battery of tests to assess your child's intellectual functioning, cognitive processing, working memory, and any potential learning disorders. Depending on the school district and if your child's school performance has been affected (failing grades), the school might have a school-based psychologist perform the testing for your child. If the school won't do this, you must arrange it yourself. Some insurance plans pay in part for these, but they can cost a couple of thousand dollars out of pocket. If testing reveals a diagnosis, the school system must abide by this documentation. Table 9.1 lists other doctoral-level providers and their degree types and specializations.

Therapists

Psychotherapists may be either doctoral-level or master's-level in a mental health or counseling profession. You'll notice different licenses and credentials when you're looking for a therapist. In Table 9.2, the variety of professions and providers that provide mental health services are listed, along with their field and level of training.

To help you find a therapist, I have provided websites of various parenting programs that list certified providers in chapter 10 and the

Table 9.1. Doctoral-Level Clinicians

Terms and Abbreviations	Meaning
PsyD (Clinical Doctorate in Psychology)	The person has graduated from a four- to five-year program focusing on psychotherapy with a one-year internship.
PhD in Clinical Psychology	The person has graduated from a doctoral program in clinical psychology. They have also completed a one-year internship and a dissertation. Many clinical psychology graduates end up as researchers but some become clinicians.
PhD in Counseling Psychology	The person has graduated from a four- to five-year program in counseling within a school of education.
Nurse Practitioner (NP)	Has completed a master's program and now, more typically, a doctoral-level nurse practitioner program. Those practicing as a psychiatric mental health nurse practitioner can provide therapy and medications.
Medical Doctor (Psychiatrist)	A psychiatrist is a medical doctor first and foremost and has done an additional training residency in psychiatry.
Doctorate in Clinical Social Work (DSW)	A relatively new type of advanced clinical training. Understand that the MSW (the master's) also qualifies people to become therapists.

Resources section. In addition, search on *Psychology Today*'s therapy finder site and filter by your insurance plan to find clinicians. Understand that like all medical services, you will probably have a patient co-pay to fulfill. These can be paid by Health Service Accounts (HSAs) that may be offered as part of your insurance plan. They range in size from $10 a session to 50 percent of the session cost. Therapists charge a range of fees for their services. In big cities now, psychotherapy sessions are $200 and more. They may be lower in other parts of the country, like $150–$175. If a provider accepts insurance, the insurance company picks up the cost, and you are only left to contribute the co-pay.

If you don't have insurance, organizations in your community and surrounding area provide sliding-scale fee services. Depending on your state, they may be called Family Service centers or Community Boards. Religiously affiliated nonprofits also offer sliding-scale services, such as Catholic Charities, Jewish Social Services, and Lutheran Social Services. Despite their affiliations, they are open to people of all faiths and do not tout a particular doctrine for recipients. If none of these

Table 9.2. Master's-Level Therapists

Terms and Abbreviations	Meaning
Master's in Social Work (MSW)	The person has graduated from a two-years master's program in social work from an accredited university.
Licensed Clinical Social Worker (LCSW)	In addition to receiving a Master's in Social Work, the provider meets state guidelines for extended practice after receiving the degree (usually two to five years) and has been supervised.
Master's in Educational Counseling (MEd)	The person has graduated from a two-year master's program in counseling located within a school of education.
Master's in Professional Counseling (MA or MS)	The person has graduated from a two-year master's program in counseling within a school of psychology.
Licensed Professional Counselor (LPC)	The person has graduated with a master's in educational or professional counseling and meets state guidelines for extended practice (typically two to five years) and has been supervised.
Marriage and Family Therapist (MFT)	The provider has graduated from a two-year master's program in marriage and family therapy.
Licensed Marriage and Family Therapist (LMFT)	In addition to graduating from a two-year master's program in marriage and family therapy, the provider meets state guidelines for extended practice after receiving the degree (usually two to five years) and has been supervised.

avenues find you a provider, type in "sliding-scale fee mental health counseling" and your city/area in a web browser to find resources.

PAYMENT FOR SERVICES

A lot of the stress with trying to manage a mental disability is the cost of treatment. Here are some options for reducing costs.

1. Start with your or your spouse's employee assistance program (EAP). To promote workplace mental health and prevent situations from deteriorating, which will then affect people's ability to do their job, many workplaces offer employee assistance programs in which therapists are available on a time-limited basis,

in some settings as many as eight sessions, for no cost. Despite the fact that these services are part of workplace benefits, the sessions are private and confidential, and occur on tele-therapy or at another location. Therefore, your supervisor, director, and colleagues will not know if you access these confidential services. Sessions are free for family members up to eight sessions. This can at least get treatment started, and if you have good results from the EAP therapist, they can often continue to see your child and family through your insurance and/or private pay.

2. Use your pediatrician as much as possible for diagnoses, medication management, and referrals.

3. If possible, put the maximum allowable in a health savings account or flexible spending account so you can use pre-tax income for deductibles, out-of-pocket expenses, and co-pays.

4. Some schools provide counseling groups and/or have therapists come into the school to provide services. Indeed, research indicates that children are more likely to receive mental health services in school than in any other public system.[9] Therefore, your child may receive individual therapy at the school, especially if she has an emotional disability.

5. Search for "Family Assessment and Planning Team" in your state and specific area. This is a multidisciplinary team of community providers from a variety of child-focused organizations and agencies that get involved in complex cases that need a lot of resources. Your child's school social worker should be able to refer you to these services.

6. For your insurance plan, pick a plan during open enrollment with the best reimbursement options for "behavioral health." Some plans provide a very minimal amount and others, such as Blue Cross Blue Shield, are more generous.

7. If you or your spouse's work setting has a "concierge" from the insurance plan to work with, use their services. They can locate more specialized referrals that are covered by your insurance plan. If possible, submit all your receipts for reimbursement through the concierge as they seem to go through this way more reliably.

8. If you have a child with high needs from their disability and low resources, you can apply for federal supplemental Social Security

benefits. This website has details on eligibility requirements and how to apply: https://www.ssa.gov/ssi/.

9. If you are ever investigated by child protective services (CPS), use it as an opportunity to get services. Of course, this is often a parent's worst nightmare, but being investigated can happen for various reasons not connected to any actual maltreatment. When you explain the mental health challenges, the toll on your family, and what services you're already engaged with, the CPS caseworker may refer you to additional services. Depending on your jurisdiction, they may authorize for prevention at sliding-scale or no cost.

10. File a Child in Need of Supervision petition with the juvenile court to gain compliance and have services paid for. See chapter 8 for a fuller discussion of the pros and cons of this practice.

SUMMARY

This chapter focuses on help-seeking across different disorders and highlights the importance of early intervention. The US mental health services system is fragmented, making it difficult to get needed services.[10] This chapter provides insights and recommendations for accessing services and resources in the mental health, social services, and criminal justice systems to support children and families in need.

Chapter 10

Parenting Interventions

This chapter homes in on interventions for parents. In some ways, that might not seem fair. Your child is the problem, why does the parent have to change? Doesn't that imply that you have done something wrong?

Not at all. Parenting a child with a mental health disability is much harder than parenting a neurotypical child, which is sufficiently challenging on its own. Additionally, children are generally unmotivated for treatment. When the subject is broached, they feel defensive, ashamed, exposed, at fault, and to blame; no wonder they wouldn't want to engage in a change process. Wouldn't that imply they were to blame? They also have cognitive limitations, which means they lack insight and have yet to develop the ability to articulate thoughts and feelings. By changing the environment, they learn to respond in different ways, and you help them progress much faster than if they were to be only involved in treatment.

In this chapter, I cover some of the current parenting programs that parents with children with mental disorders find appealing and that might cross-cut disorders. Indeed, most, except for Lives in the Balance, which is for "explosive" children, are designed for parents of any child, not specifically for mental disorder. Most do a nice job of balancing both attachment and behavior. I'll roughly group them according to developmental stage of the child. Recognize that many of the popular parenting programs have not been studied.

INFANT/BABY STAGE

Written for the infant and baby stage, *Raising the Spirited Baby* guides
parents of children with temperament challenges. Each chapter in this
book has discussed temperament's role in the development of the disorder. Temperament provides the foundation for personality. It includes
biologically driven qualities observed from infancy and moderately stable across the life span and in different contexts.[1] Temperament involves
the following aspects: intensity, sensitivity, alertness, regularity, activity
level, social activity, persistence, adaptability, and seriousness.

Touted as covering parenting of children from babies to school age,
Now Say This also balances warmth and attunement, and limit-setting
and reality. The contention of authors Heather Tuegeon and Julie Wright
is that limit setting must occur in the context of a positive relationship.

They warn against certain parenting go-tos:

- Judgement and shaming: "What's wrong with you?"
- Making dismissive comments: "It's not a big deal."
- Harshness: "You're driving me up a wall. How many times do I
  have to tell you?"
- Trying to cut off communication: "Because I said so." "No
  means no."
- Threatening and punishing: "Do you want to go to time-out?"
- Comparing: "Look how nicely your cousin is sitting there."

Their three-step process is:

1. Attunement, which involves empathy, allowing space for the child
   to share feelings and perspective, and finding some way to agree
   and align: "That would be so fun to shop for the party dress now."
2. Use the "Iceberg Analogy," digging deeper than the child's behavior and going for the underlying reasons: "You're getting tired
   after being out all this time."
3. Dealing with reality ("Rex can't play today after school") and
   limit setting with a brief reason provided ("We have to leave now
   to get home before your sister arrives").

PRESCHOOL

Aha Parenting (https://www.ahaparenting.com) is an approach by Dr. Laura Markham that focuses on child feelings and attachment in the parent-child relationship as a vehicle to influence child behavior.[2] Dr. Markham formulated the approach for parents of "normal" children, but she contends that a parent would work the same way with a child diagnosed with a mental health disorder, although perhaps more intensely.[3]

Three basic principles undergird the work. First parents must focus on regulating their own emotions. It's easy to get irritated and activated yourself when your child is noisy, disruptive, and infuriating; it may not be possible to stay regulated all the time, so often the best you can do is to keep your emotions in tap and present a neutral demeanor. Dr. Markham contends that the child learns emotional regulation from the parent.

Second, a strong parent-child connection gives the parent influence with their child. This means showing empathy for what they're going through: "I can see how frustrated you are that Rex isn't available to play this afternoon. You like spending time with him so much." Take it as a good sign if your child cries in response as this means release from an overwrought system.

Third, coach instead of controlling (emotion-coaching), meaning if the parent can help their child with "big emotions," the child will learn to self-regulate. Once kids can manage their emotions, they can manage their behavior. Dr. Markham promotes roughhousing and silliness as a way to discharge anxiety, bond in a physical way with children, and show them they're still loveable. Another part of connection is having "special playtime" in a fifteen-minute slot each day with just one child at a time. The website lists a directory of trained clinicians: https://www.ahaparenting.com/coaches-directory, and parenting classes are also available.

SCHOOL AGE

Love and Logic

Love and Logic is geared toward school-age children[4] and teens.[5] The main point of the system is that your child experiences the consequences of their own choices and decisions rather than imposing your will, which often leads to child resentment. If a consequence happens because of a child's actions, such as a poor grade or a traffic ticket, rather than scolding, we say something like, "Oh, that's too bad. That's a bummer to have to pay that ticket now." As a result, they experience their own consequences, directing their anger at themselves rather than railing against you. In this way, growth and maturity result.

1-2-3 Magic

1-2-3 Magic centers around a variant of time-out but expands beyond this technique into problem-solving, rewards, and creating a positive family environment.[6] In my experience, the 1-2-3 technique is more productive for families than traditional time-out. Additionally, it's relatively easy to learn and implement because it centers on one technique.

In 1-2-3 Magic, when the child first makes an undesirable behavior (let's say, starting to become rude), the parent warns "one." If the child continues with the onerous behavior, the parent warns, "two." If the child continues, the parent says, "Okay, that's three. Go to your room."

Although a kid's room still has plenty to do, and a pure behaviorist might object that a time-out should be free from any reinforcement, the main point here is to interrupt a negative interaction at low levels rather than waiting for it to escalate. It also offers a chance for everyone to regroup and reset with no need to revisit the topic. For kids with certain challenges, apologizing or admitting they're wrong triggers defensiveness and potential further escalation. Your public library should have a copy of the video, which is an accessible way to grasp the model's essential features.

Lives in the Balance

Lives in the Balance is an approach developed by clinical psychologist Dr. Ross Greene that focuses on understanding and addressing the underlying skills and triggers behind a child's challenging behavior, rather than labeling it as willful misbehavior.[7] Rather than blaming the child or considering their behavior intentional, the approach views misbehavior as a signal that the child is struggling and needs support. Parents are encouraged to "swim upstream" and identify the triggers that led to out-of-control behavior. The assumption is that the child lacks the necessary skills to manage the situation effectively. For instance, emotional regulation comprises impulse control, self-soothing, and problem-solving.

The approach emphasizes collaborative problem-solving between parents and children to find mutually agreeable solutions to unsolved problems. When discussing a specific situation with the child, parents aim to have the conversation when the child has calmed down and is more receptive to dialogue. Instead of lecturing or imposing solutions, parents show patience and curiosity, allowing the child to express their concerns and contribute ideas for resolving the problem. Both parents and children share their perspectives and work toward finding a mutually agreeable solution.

The Lives in the Balance approach provides resources such as videotapes, podcast episodes, and parenting classes on their website to demonstrate the model: https://livesinthebalance.org/. Support is offered through a moderated Facebook group called The B Team, where parents can connect and receive guidance. The approach differentiates between Plan A (a unilateral solution imposed by the parent), Plan B (collaborative problem-solving), and Plan C (setting aside certain expectations temporarily due to the child's inability to meet them). Compared to the decades of research on parent training approaches, research is at the beginning stages for Lives in the Balance. The couple of randomized controlled trials show that the Lives in the Balance approach was as effective as parent training for oppositional behaviors in children[8] and in reducing child and adolescent severe irritability compared to usual care.[9]

HELP FOR PARENTS AND FAMILIES

Raising a child with a disability can be a source of immense stress and may contribute to clinical depression. Individual treatment for yourself might be beneficial if hopelessness and helplessness persist. It also might be indicated if you've had trauma from childhood, particularly in the context of your family of origin, that you want to avoid bringing into your current family. Free parenting support resources are offered in the Resources section.

Some parents turn to substances to cope with the extreme stress of family life. Alcoholics Anonymous self-help groups and treatment-based approaches (the Minnesota model) have predominated in the substance-abuse treatment field. The AA stance is that alcohol is a progressive disease and that, due to underlying vulnerabilities, certain people, called alcoholics, can only strive for total abstinence. Because of the lure of alcohol, only a "higher power," defined by each individual, even if only the "power of the group," can help "restore people to sanity" when they are lost in the grip of alcohol. AA approaches are also called "twelve-step" as there are a series of steps that members work under the guidance of a sponsor. A sponsor has achieved a significant amount of time in sobriety. While AA self-help groups offer several advantages, the model doesn't resonate with everyone. Other self-help groups for addictions exist, and many now hold meetings online. Total abstinence, like the AA goal, is promoted in some (e.g., Women for Sobriety), but others have more flexibility around goals. See the Resources section at the end of the book.

The presence of the disability and the constant efforts required to manage it can significantly impact the entire family. As a result, relationships between parents may become strained, and there are usually different parenting styles. One person assumes the role of primary caregiver while the partner either withdraws or gets angry. Parenting a child with high needs demands great sensitivity and can be challenging to sustain consistently. The demands placed on parents to meet these needs can exacerbate existing cracks in the relationship. Consequently, parents often feel exhausted and lacking in support.

Couples counseling can be a viable option for parents in such situations. It is not necessary for counseling to be a long-term commitment; even a relatively brief period of eight to twelve sessions can be enormously beneficial for most individuals. To maximize the effectiveness of therapy, I recommend finding a therapist who specializes in couples work and has extensive experience in this area. Given the intricacies of couple dynamics, the therapist must operate from a well-established framework offering coherent theories on couple dynamics and interventions that have been documented and practiced over many years. While not all have undergone rigorous research scrutiny (e.g., Imago Therapy), most have empirical support. The list in Resources includes websites where you can find trained providers and self-help resources associated with their programs.

One last note about families: A child with a mental disorder requires much in the way of family resources, and often siblings feel neglected and resentful, which may lead to other problems.[10] As much as possible, ensure each child gets the attention they need.

SUMMARY

This chapter emphasized the unique challenges of parenting children with mental health disabilities. By changing the family environment and utilizing effective strategies, parents can help their children make a better adjustment. This chapter has presented several parenting programs that are applicable across different disorders and developmental stages. Additionally, the chapter recognizes the strain on family members, siblings, and relationships between parents and offers resources to navigate these challenges. Overall, by being empowered with information and support, you can maximize the well-being of your family.

Notes

INTRODUCTION

1. Daniel G. Whitney and Mark D. Peterson, "US National and State-Level Prevalence of Mental Health Disorders and Disparities of Mental Health Care Use in Children," *JAMA Pediatrics* 173, no. 4 (2019): 389–91, https://doi.org/10.1001/jamapediatrics.2018.5399.

2. American Psychiatric Association, *Diagnostic and Statistical Manual of Mental Disorders,* 5th ed., text revision (DSM-5-TR) (Washington, DC: American Psychiatric Association, 2022).

3. Jacqueline Corcoran and Joseph Walsh, *Clinical Assessment and Diagnosis in Social Work Practice*, 4th ed. (New York: Oxford University Press, 2022).

4. Anne Harrington, *Mind Fixers: Psychiatry's Troubled Search for the Biology of Mental Illness* (New York: W.W. Norton & Company, 2020).

5. Harrington, *Mind Fixers*.

6. Gardiner Harris, "Drug Maker Told Studies Would Aid It, Papers Say," *New York Times*, March 19, 2009.

7. Gardiner Harris, "Research Center Tied to Drug Company," *New York Times*, November 24, 2008.

8. Gardiner Harris and Benedict Carey, "Researchers Fail to Reveal Full Drug Pay," *New York Times*, June 8, 2008.

CHAPTER 1

1. Melissa L. Danielson, et al., "Prevalence of Parent-Reported ADHD Diagnosis and Associated Treatment Among U.S. Children and Adolescents,

2016," *Journal of Clinical Child and Adolescent Psychology* 47, no. (2, (2018): 199–212, http://doi.org/10.1080/15374416.2017.1417860.

2. Stephen Hinshaw, "Attention Deficit Hyperactivity Disorder (ADHD): Controversy, Developmental Mechanisms, and Multiple Levels of Analysis," *Annual Review of Clinical Psychology* 14 (2018): 291–316, https://doi.org/10.1146/annurev-clinpsy-050817-084917.

3. Danielson et al., "Prevalence of Parent-Reported ADHD Diagnosis and Associated Treatment."

4. Susana N. Visser et al., "Demographic Differences Among a National Sample of US Youth with Behavioral Disorders," *Clinical Pediatrics* 55, no. 14 (2016): 1358–62, https://doi.org/10.1177/0009922815623229.

5. American Psychiatric Association, *Diagnostic and Statistical Manual of Mental Disorders*, 5th ed., text revision (DSM-5-TR) (Washington, DC: American Psychiatric Association).

6. *Diagnostic and Statistical Manual of Mental Disorders.*

7. Thomas E. Brown and William J. McMullen, "Attention Deficit Disorders and Sleep/Arousal Disturbance," *Annals of the New York Academy of Sciences Journal* 931 (2001): 271–86, https://doi.org/10.1111/j.1749-6632.2001.tb05784.x.

8. Jacqueline Corcoran et al., "Parents of Children with Attention Deficit/Hyperactivity Disorder: A Meta-Synthesis, Part I," *Child and Adolescent Social Work Journal* 34 (2017): 281–335, DOI: 10.1007/s10560-016-0465-1; Jacqueline Corcoran et al., "Parents of Children with Attention Deficit/Hyperactivity Disorder: A Meta-Synthesis, Part II," *Child and Adolescent Social Work Journal* 34 (2017): 337–48, DOI: 10.1007/s10560-017-0497-1.

9. Tycho J. Dekkers et al., "Meta-Analysis: Which Components of Parent Training Work for Children with Attention-Deficit/Hyperactivity Disorder?," *Journal of the American Academy of Child & Adolescent Psychiatry* 61, no. 4 (2022): 478–94, https://doi.org/10.1016/j.jaac.2021.06.015.

10. James R. D. Tucker and Christopher W. Hobson, "A Systematic Review of Longitudinal Studies Investigating the Association Between Early Life Maternal Depression and Offspring ADHD," *Journal of Attention Disorders* 26, no. 9 (2022): 1167–86, http://doi.org/10.1177/10870547211063642; Anne Wüstner et al., "Risk and Protective Factors for the Development of ADHD Symptoms in Children and Adolescents: Results of the Longitudinal BELLA Study," *PLOS One* 14, no. 3 (2019), https://doi.org/10.1371/journal.pone.0214412.

11. Corcoran et al., "Parents of Children with Attention Deficit/Hyperactivity Disorder: Part I."

12. Katherine A. Johnson, Jan R. Wiersema, and Jonna Kuntsi, "What Would Karl Popper Say? Are Current Psychological Theories of ADHD

Falsifiable?," *Behavioral and Brain Functions* 5, no. 15 (2009): 1–11, https://doi.org/10.1186/1744-9081-5-15.

13. Heledd Hart et al., "Meta-Analysis of Functional Magnetic Resonance Imaging Studies of Inhibition and Attention in Attention-Deficit Hyperactivity Disorder: Exploring Task-Specific, Stimulant Medication, and Age Effects," *Journal of American Medical Association Psychiatry* 70, no. 2 (2013): 185–98, https://doi.org/10.1001/jamapsychiatry.2013.277.

14. M. Uchida et al., "The Heritability of ADHD in Children of ADHD Parents: A Post-Hoc Analysis of Longitudinal Data," *Journal of Attention Disorders* 27, no. 3 (2023): 250–57, https://doi.org/10.1177/10870547221136251.

15. Benjamin M. Neale et al., "Meta-Analysis of Genome-Wide Association Studies of Attention-Deficit/Hyperactivity Disorder," *Journal of the American Academy of Child and Adolescent Psychiatry* 49, no. 9 (2010): 884–97, https://doi.org/10.1016/j.jaac.2010.06.008.

16. Ian R. Gizer, Courtney Ficks, and Irwin D. Waldman, "Candidate Gene Studies of ADHD: A Meta-Analytic Review," *Human Genetics* 126 (2009): 51–90, https://doi.org/10.1007/s00439-009-0694-x.

17. Irene Tung et al., "Patterns of Comorbidity Among Girls with ADHD: A Meta-Analysis," *Pediatrics* 138, no. 4 (2016), https://doi.org/10.1542/peds.2016-0430.

18. Elis Haan et al., "Prenatal Smoking, Alcohol and Caffeine Exposure and Maternal-Reported Attention Deficit Hyperactivity Disorder Symptoms in Childhood: Triangulation of Evidence Using Negative Control and Polygenic Risk Score Analyses," *Addiction* 117, no. 5 (2022): 1458–71, https://doi.org/10.1111/add.15746.

19. L. C. Chen et al., "Association of Parental Depression with Offspring Attention Deficit Hyperactivity Disorder and Autism Spectrum Disorder: A Nationwide Birth Cohort Study," *Journal of Affective Disorders* 277 (2020): 109–14, https://doi.org/10.1016/j.jad.2020.07.059.

20. C. H. Hemmingsen et al., "Maternal Use of Hormonal Contraception and Risk of Childhood ADHD: A Nationwide Population-Based Cohort Study," *European Journal of Epidemiology* 35, no. 9 (2020): 795–805, https://doi.org/10.1007/s10654-020-00673-w.

21. Jae H. Kim et al., "Environmental Risk Factors, Protective Factors, and Peripheral Biomarkers for ADHD: An Umbrella Review," *The Lancet* 7, no. 11 (2020): 955–70, https://doi.org/10.1016/S2215-0366(20)30312-6.

22. Won-Jun Choi et al., "Blood Lead, Parental Marital Status and the Risk of Attention-Deficit/Hyperactivity Disorder in Elementary School Children: A Longitudinal Study," *Psychiatry Research* 236 (2016): 42–46, https://doi.org/10.1016/j.psychres.2016.01.002.

23. Maryse F. Bouchard et al., "Attention-Deficit/ Hyperactivity Disorder and Urinary Metabolites of Organophosphate Pesticides," *Pediatrics* 125, no. 6 (2010): 1270–77, https://doi.org/10.1542/peds.2009-3058.

24. Danielson et al., "Prevalence of Parent-Reported ADHD Diagnosis and Associated Treatment."

25. Michaela M. Cordova et al., "Attention-Deficit/Hyperactivity Disorder: Restricted Phenotypes Prevalence, Comorbidity, and Polygenic Risk Sensitivity in the ABCD Baseline Cohort," *Journal of the American Academy of Child & Adolescent Psychiatry* 61, no. 10 (2022): 1273–84, https://doi.org/10.1016/j.jaac.2022.03.030.

26. Daniel F. Connor, Jennifer Steeber, and Keith McBurnett, "A Review of Attention-Deficit/Hyperactivity Disorder Complicated by Symptoms of Oppositional Defiant Disorder or Conduct Disorder," *Journal of Developmental and Behavioral Pediatrics* 31 (2010): 427–40, https://doi.org/10.1097/DBP.0b013e3181e121bd.

27. Sean Perrin, Patrick Smith, and William Yule, "Practitioner Review: The Assessment and Treatment of Post-Traumatic Stress Disorder in Children and Adolescents," *Journal of Child Psychology and Psychiatry and Allied Disciplines* 41, no. 3, (2000), 277–89.

28. Jill Furzer, Elizabeth Dhuey, and Audrey Laporte, "ADHD Misdiagnosis: Causes and Mitigators," *Health Economics* 31, no. 9 (2022): 1926–53, https://doi.org/10.1002/hec.4555.

29. Lily Hechtman and Elizabeth Owens, "The Berkeley Girls with ADHD Longitudinal Study," in *Attention Deficit Hyperactivity Disorder: Adult Outcome and Its Predictors* (New York: Oxford University Press, 2017), 179–229.

30. Meredith Bergey et al., "Mapping Mental Health Inequalities: The Intersecting Effects of Gender, Race, Class, and Ethnicity on ADHD Diagnosis," *Sociology of Health & Illness* 44, no. 3 (2022): 604–23, doi:10.1111/1467-9566.13443.

31. Paul L. Morgan et al., "Racial and Ethnic Disparities in ADHD Diagnosis from Kindergarten to Eighth Grade," *Pediatrics* 132, no. 1 (2013): 85–93, https://doi.org/10.1542/peds.2012-2390.

32. Amy Glasofer, Catherine Dingley, and Andrew T. Reyes, "Medication Decision Making Among African American Caregivers of Children with ADHD: A Review of Literature," *Journal of Attention Disorders* 25, no. 12 (2021): 1687–98, https://doi.org/10.1177/1087054720930783.

33. Bergey et al., "Mapping Mental Health Inequalities."

34. Timothy J. Layton et al., "Attention Deficit–Hyperactivity Disorder and Month of School Enrollment," *New England Journal of Medicine* 379, no. 22 (2018): 2122–30, https://doi.org/10.1056/NEJMoa1806828.

35. Monica Shaw et al., "A Systematic Review and Analysis of Long-Term Outcomes in Attention Deficit Hyperactivity Disorder: Effects of Treatment

and Non-Treatment," *BMC Medicine* 10 (2012): 99, http://doi.org/10.1186/1741-7015-10-99.

36. Shaw et al., "Long-Term Outcomes in Attention Deficit Hyperactivity Disorder."

37. Danielson et al., "Prevalence of Parent-Reported ADHD Diagnosis and Associated Treatment"; James G. Waxmonsky et al., "A Commercial Insurance Claims Analysis of Correlates of Behavioral Therapy Use Among Children with ADHD," *Psychiatric Services* 70, no. 12 (2019): 1116–22, https://doi.org/10.1176/appi.ps.201800473.

38. Hinshaw, "Attention Deficit Hyperactivity Disorder (ADHD)."

39. Benjamin J. Lovett and Jason M. Nelson, "Systematic Review: Educational Accommodations for Children and Adolescents with Attention-Deficit/Hyperactivity Disorder," *Journal of the American Academy of Child and Adolescent Psychiatry* 60, no. 4 (2021), 448–57.

40. Lovett and Nelson, "Educational Accommodations for Children and Adolescents with Attention-Deficit/Hyperactivity Disorder."

41. Gregory A. Fabiano and Kellina Pyle, "Best Practices in School Mental Health for Attention-Deficit/Hyperactivity Disorder: A Framework for Intervention," *School Mental Health* 11, no. 1 (2019): 72–91, https://doi.org/10.1007/s12310-018-9267-2.

42. Gregory A. Fabiano et al., "Special Education for Children with ADHD: Services Received and a Comparison to Children with ADHD in General Education," *School Mental Health* 14, no. 4 (2022): 818–30.

43. Mark L. Wolraich et al., "Clinical Practice Guideline for the Diagnosis, Evaluation, and Treatment of Attention-Deficit/Hyperactivity Disorder in Children and Adolescents," *Pediatrics* 144, no. 4 (2019): e20192528, https://doi.org/10.1542/peds.2019-2528.

44. Laurence L. Greenhill et al., "Trajectories of Growth Associated with Long-Term Stimulant Medication in the Multimodal Treatment Study of Attention-Deficit/Hyperactivity Disorder," *Journal of the American Academy of Child & Adolescent Psychiatry* 59, no. 8 (2020): 978–89, https://doi.org/10.1016/j.jaac.2019.06.019.

45. Walt Karniski, *ADHD Medication: Does It Work and Is It Safe?* (Lanham, MD: Rowman & Littlefield, 2022).

46. Daniel Safer, "Recent Trends in Stimulant Usage," *Journal of Attention Disorders* 20, no. 6 (2016): 471–77, https://doi.org/10.1177/1087054715605915.

47. Karniski, *ADHD Medication.*

48. James Swanson et al., "Evidence, Interpretation, and Qualification from Multiple Reports of Long-Term Outcomes in the Multimodal Treatment Study of Children with ADHD (MTA): Part I: Executive Summary," *Journal of Attention Disorders* 12, no. 1 (2008): 4–14, https://doi.org/10.1177/1087054708319345.

49. Mark Olfson, Steven Marcus, and George Wan, "Stimulant Dosing for Children with ADHD: A Medical Claims Analysis," *Journal of the American Academy of Child & Adolescent Psychiatry* 48, no. 1 (2009): 51–59, https://doi.org/10.1097/CHI.0b013e31818b1c8f.

50. Wolraich et al., "Diagnosis, Evaluation, and Treatment of Attention-Deficit/Hyperactivity Disorder in Children and Adolescents."

51. Samuele Cortese et al., "Comparative Efficacy and Tolerability of Medications for Attention-Deficit Hyperactivity Disorder in Children, Adolescents, and Adults: A Systematic Review and Network Meta-Analysis," *The Lancet* 5, no. 9 (2018): 727–38, https://doi.org/10.1016/S2215-0366(18)30269-4.

52. Salima Punja et al., "Amphetamines for Attention Deficit Hyperactivity Disorder (ADHD) in Children and Adolescents," *Cochrane Database of Systematic Reviews* 2 (2016): 471–77, https://doi.org/10.1177/1087054715605915.

53. Corcoran et al., "Parents of Children with Attention Deficit/Hyperactivity Disorder: Part I."

54. Karniski, *ADHD Medication.*

55. Greenhill et al., "Trajectories of Growth Associated with Long-Term Stimulant Medication."

56. Karniski, *ADHD Medication.*

57. Steven W. Evans, Julie S. Owens, and Nora Bunford, "Evidence-Based Psychosocial Treatments for Children and Adolescents with Attention-Deficit/Hyperactivity Disorder," *Journal of Clinical Child and Adolescent Psychology* 43, no. 4 (2014): 527–51, https://doi.org/10.1080/15374416.2013.850700.

58. Dekkers et al., "The Importance of Parental Knowledge in the Association between ADHD Symptomatology and Related Domains of Impairment," *European Journal of Child Adolescent Psychiatry* 30, no. 4 (2021): 657–69, https://doi.org/10.1007/s00787-020-01579-4.

59. Wolraich et al., "Diagnosis, Evaluation, and Treatment of Attention-Deficit/Hyperactivity Disorder in Children and Adolescents."

60. Tycho J. Dekkers et al., "Decision-Making Deficits in Adolescent Boys with and without Attention-Deficit/Hyperactivity Disorder (ADHD): An Experimental Assessment of Associated Mechanisms," *Journal of Abnormal Child Psychology* 48, no. 4 (2020): 495–510, https://doi.org/10.1007/s10802-019-00613-7.

61. Corcoran et al., "Parents of Children with Attention Deficit/Hyperactivity Disorder: Part I"; Corcoran et al., "Parents of Children with Attention Deficit/Hyperactivity Disorder: Part II."

62. Francesco Craig et al., "A Systematic Review of Coping Strategies in Parents of Children with Attention Deficit Hyperactivity Disorder (ADHD)," *Research in Developmental Disabilities* 98 (2020): 103571, https://doi.org/10.1016/j.ridd.2020.103571.

63. Zheng Chang et al., "Stimulant ADHD Medication and Risk for Substance Abuse," *Journal of Child Psychology and Psychiatry* 55 (2014): 878–85, https://doi-org.proxy.library.upenn.edu/10.1111/jcpp.12164.

64. Eugenia Chan, Jason M. Fogler, and Paul G. Hammerness, "Treatment of Attention-Deficit/Hyperactivity Disorder in Adolescents: A Systematic Review," *Journal of American Medical Association* 315, no. 8 (2016): 1997–2008, https://doi.org/10.1001/jama.2016.5453.

65. Gal Shoval et al., "Evaluation of Attention-Deficit/Hyperactivity Disorder Medications, Externalizing Symptoms, and Suicidality in Children," *JAMA Network Open* 4, no. 6 (2021), https://doi.org/10.1001/jamanetworkopen.2021.11342.

CHAPTER 2

1. American Psychiatric Association, *Diagnostic and Statistical Manual of Mental Disorders* (DSM-5-TR) (Washington, DC: American Psychiatric Association, 2022).

2. Michelle M. Hughes et al., "The Prevalence and Characteristics of Children with Profound Autism, 15 Sites, United States, 2000–2016," *Public Health Reports*, 2023, 003335492311635, https://doi.org/10.1177/00333549231163551.

3. *In a Different Key: The Story of Autism*, PBS, 2013, https://www.pbs.org/show/different-key/.

4. "Identity-First Language," Autistic Self Advocacy Network, n.d., https://autisticadvocacy.org/about-asan/identity-first-language/.

5. Emily Ramsey et al., "Autism Spectrum Disorder Prevalence Rates in the United States: Methodologies, Challenges, and Implications for Individual States," *Journal of Developmental and Physical Disabilities* 28, no. 1 (2016): 803–20, https://doi.org/10.1007/s10882-016-9510-4.

6. "Autism and Developmental Disabilities Monitoring (ADDM) Network," Centers for Disease Control, n.d., https://www.cdc.gov/ncbddd/autism/pdf/ADDM-Community-Report-SY2020-h.pdf.

7. Matthew J. Maenner et al., "Prevalence and Characteristics of Autism Spectrum Disorder Among Children Aged 8 Years—Autism and Developmental Disabilities Monitoring Network, 11 Sites, United States, 2020," *MMWR, Surveillance Summaries* 72, no. 2 (2023): 1–14, https://doi.org/10.15585/mmwr.ss7202a1.

8. Rebecca E. Rosenberg et al., "Factors Affecting Age at Initial Autism Spectrum Disorder Diagnosis in a National Survey," *Autism Research and Treatment* (2011): 1–11, https://doi.org/10.1155/2011/874619.

9. Maya Matheis et al., "Factors Related to Parental Age of First Concern in Toddlers with Autism Spectrum Disorder," *Developmental Neurorehabilitation* 20, no. 4 (2016): 228–35, https://doi.org/10.1080/17518423.2016.1211186.

10. Amy M. Daniels and David S. Mandell, "Explaining Differences in Age at Autism Spectrum Disorder Diagnosis: A Critical Review," *Autism* 18, no. 5 (2013): 583–97, https://doi.org/10.1177/1362361313480277.

11. Natacha D. Emerson, Holly E. Morrell, and Cameron Neece, "Predictors of Age of Diagnosis for Children with Autism Spectrum Disorder: The Role of a Consistent Source of Medical Care, Race, and Condition Severity," *Journal of Autism and Developmental Disorders* 46, no. 1 (2016): 127–38, https://doi.org/10.1007/s10803-015-2555-x.

12. Nicolas Deconinck, Marie Soncarrieu, and Bernard Dan, "Toward Better Recognition of Early Predictors for Autism Spectrum Disorders," *Pediatric Neurology* 49, no. 4 (2013): 225–31, https://doi.org/10.1016/j.pediatrneurol.2013.05.012.

13. Claire Hathorn et al., "Impact of Adherence to Best Practice Guidelines on the Diagnostic and Assessment Services for Autism Spectrum Disorder," *Journal of Autism and Developmental Disorders* 44, no. 8 (2014): 1859–66, https://doi.org/10.1007/s10803-014-2057-2.

14. Beata Tick et al., "Heritability of Autism Spectrum Disorders: A Meta-Analysis of Twin Studies," *Journal of Child Psychology and Psychiatry* 57, no. 5 (2016): 585–95, https://doi.org/10.1111/jcpp.12499.

15. Neil Risch et al., "Familial Recurrence of Autism Spectrum Disorder: Evaluating Genetic and Environmental Contributions," *American Journal of Psychiatry* 171, no. 11 (2014): 1206–13, https://doi.org/10.1176/appi.ajp.2014.13101359.

16. Xiao Ji et al., "Increased Burden of Deleterious Variants in Essential Genes in Autism Spectrum Disorder," *Proceedings of the National Academy of Sciences* 113, no. 52 (2016): 15054–59, https://doi.org/10.1073/pnas.1613195113.

17. Esther Vierck and Jeremy M. Silverman, "Brief Report: Phenotypic Differences and Their Relationship to Paternal Age and Gender in Autism Spectrum Disorder," *Journal of Autism and Developmental Disorders* 45 (2015): 1915–24, https://doi.org/10.1007/s10803-014-2346-9.

18. Amirhossein Modabbernia, Eva Velthorst, and Abraham Reichenberg, "Environmental Risk Factors for Autism: An Evidence-Based Review of Systematic Reviews and Meta-Analyses," *Molecular Autism* 8, no. 1 (2017), https://doi.org/10.1186/s13229-017-0121-4.

19. D. A. Rossignol, S. J. Genuis, and R. E. Frye, "Environmental Toxicants and Autism Spectrum Disorders: A Systematic Review," *Translational Psychiatry* 4, no. 2 (2014), https://doi.org/10.1038/tp.2014.4.

20. Amirhossein Modabbernia, Eva Velthorst, and Abraham Reichenberg, "Environmental Risk Factors for Autism: An Evidence-Based Review of Systematic Reviews and Meta-Analyses," *Molecular Autism* 8, no. 1 (2017), https://doi.org/10.1186/s13229-017-0121-4.

21. Michelle Ng et al., "Environmental Factors Associated with Autism Spectrum Disorder: A Scoping Review for the Years 2003–2013," *Health Promotion and Chronic Disease Prevention in Canada* 37, no. 1 (2017): 1–23, https://doi.org/10.24095/hpcdp.37.1.01.

22. Amaria Baghdadli et al., "Developmental Trajectories of Adaptive Behaviors from Early Childhood to Adolescence in a Cohort of 152 Children with Autism Spectrum Disorders," *Journal of Autism and Developmental Disorders* 42 (2012): 1314–25, https://doi.org/10.1007/s10803-011-1357-z.

23. Nina Jamilette Hidalgo, Laura Lee McIntyre, and Ellen Hawley McWhirter, "Sociodemographic Differences in Parental Satisfaction with an Autism Spectrum Disorder Diagnosis," *Journal of Intellectual and Developmental Disability* 40, no. 2 (2015): 147–55, https://doi.org/10.3109/13668250.2014.994171.

24. Abir K. Bekhet, Norah L. Johnson, and Jaclene A. Zauszniewski, "Resilience in Family Members of Persons with Autism Spectrum Disorder: A Review of the Literature," *Issues in Mental Health Nursing* 33, no. 10 (2012): 650–56, https://doi.org/10.3109/01612840.2012.671441.

25. A. Sam et al., "Selecting an Evidence-Based Practice," AFIRM, 2022, https://afirm.fpg.unc.edu/selecting-evidence-based-practice.

26. Zehra Hangül and Ali Evren Tufan, "Use of Complementary and Alternative Therapies in Autism Spectrum Disorder," *Psikiyatride Güncel Yaklaşımlar* 14, no. 2 (2022): 165–73, https://doi.org/10.18863/pgy.935207.

27. Brian Reichow, "Overview of Meta-Analyses on Early Intensive Behavioral Intervention for Young Children with Autism Spectrum Disorders," *Journal of Autism and Developmental Disorders* 42 (2012): 512–20, https://doi.org/10.1007/s10803-011-1218-9.

28. A. Sam and AFIRM Team, "Prompting," AFIRM, 2015, http://afirm.fpg.unc.edu/prompting.

29. Elizabeth DeVita-Raeburn and Spectrum, "Is the Most Common Therapy for Autism Cruel?," *The Atlantic*, August 12, 2016, https://www.theatlantic.com/health/archive/2016/08/aba-autism-controversy/495272/.

30. Inalegwu P. Oono, Emma J. Honey, and Helen McConachie, "Parent-Mediated Early Intervention for Young Children with Autism Spectrum Disorders (ASD)," *Cochrane Database of Systematic Reviews* 4 (2013), https://doi.org/10.1002/14651858.cd009774.pub2.

31. A. Sam and AFIRM Team, "Visual Supports," AFIRM, 2015, http://afirm.fpg.unc.edu/visual-supports.

32. S. Nowell et al., "Augmentative & Alternative Communication," AFIRM, 2022, https://afirm.fpg.unc.edu/augmentative-alternative-communication.

33. A. Sam and AFIRM Team, "Social Narratives," AFIRM, 2015, http://afirm.fpg.unc.edu/social-narratives.

34. Carol Gray and Barry M. Prizant, *The New Social Story Book* (Arlington, TX: Future Horizons, 2015).

35. Jacquelyn A. Gates, Erin Kang, and Matthew D. Lerner, "Efficacy of Group Social Skills Interventions for Youth with Autism Spectrum Disorder: A Systematic Review and Meta-Analysis," *Clinical Psychology Review* 52 (2017): 164–81, https://doi.org/10.1016/j.cpr.2017.01.006.

36. N. Garrity et al., "DNEA Resource Guides for Professionals. Supporting Social Skills," Delaware Network for Excellence in Autism, https://www.delawareautismnetwork.org/wp-content/uploads/2023/01/Supporting-Social-Skills.pdf.

37. Christophe Maïano et al., "Prevalence of School Bullying Among Youth with Autism Spectrum Disorders: A Systematic Review and Meta-Analysis," *Autism Research* 9, no. 6 (2015): 601–15, https://doi.org/10.1002/aur.1568.

38. Meng-Chuan Lai et al., "Prevalence of Co-Occurring Mental Health Diagnoses in the Autism Population: A Systematic Review and Meta-Analysis," *The Lancet Psychiatry* 6, no. 10 (2019): 819–29, https://doi.org/10.1016/s2215-0366(19)30289-5.

39. Christoph U. Correll et al., "Efficacy and Acceptability of Pharmacological, Psychosocial, and Brain Stimulation Interventions in Children and Adolescents with Mental Disorders: An Umbrella Review," *World Psychiatry* 20, no. 2 (2021): 244–75, https://doi.org/10.1002/wps.20881.

40. Kylie Hillman et al., *Interventions for Anxiety in Mainstream School-Aged Children with Autism Spectrum Disorder: A Systematic Review* (Hoboken, NJ: John Wiley & Sons, 2020).

41. Rae Thomas et al., "Parent-Child Interaction Therapy: A Meta-Analysis," *Pediatrics* 140, no. 3 (2017), https://doi.org/10.1542/peds.2017-0352.

42. Michelle A. Ward, Jennifer Theule, and Kristene Cheung, "Parent–Child Interaction Therapy for Child Disruptive Behaviour Disorders: A Meta-Analysis," *Child & Youth Care Forum* 45, no. 5 (2016): 675–90, https://doi.org/10.1007/s10566-016-9350-5.

43. Jeanne M. Madden et al. "Psychotropic Medication Use Among Insured Children with Autism Spectrum Disorder," *Journal of Autism and Developmental Disorders* 47, no. 1 (2017): 144–54, doi:10.1007/s10803-016-2946-7.

44. Jane R. Schubart, Fabian Camacho, and Douglas Leslie, "Psychotropic Medication Trends Among Children and Adolescents with Autism Spectrum Disorder in the Medicaid Program," *Autism: The International Journal of Research and Practice* 18, no. 6 (2014): 631–37, https://doi.org/10.1177/1362361313497537.

45. Donna Spencer et al., "Psychotropic Medication Use and Polypharmacy in Children with Autism Spectrum Disorders," *Pediatrics* 132, no. 5 (2013), 833–40, https://doi.org/10.1542/peds.2012-3774d.

46. Rosanna Breaux et al., "Systematic Review and Meta-Analysis: Pharmacological and Nonpharmacological Interventions for Persistent Nonepisodic Irritability," *Journal of the American Academy of Child and Adolescent Psychiatry* 62, no. 3 (2023), 318–34, https://doi.org/10.1016/j.jaac.2022.05.012.

47. Vinod S. Bhatara, Bettina Bernstein, and Sheeba Fazili, "Complementary and Integrative Treatments of Aggressiveness/Emotion Dysregulation: Associated with Disruptive Disorders and Disruptive Mood Dysregulation Disorder," *Child and Adolescent Psychiatric Clinics of North America* 32, no. 2 (2023): 297–315, https://doi.org/10.1016/j.chc.2022.08.010.

48. Jason F. Earle, "An Introduction to the Psychopharmacology of Children and Adolescents with Autism Spectrum Disorder," *Journal of Child and Adolescent Psychiatric Nursing* 29, no. 2 (2016): 62–71, https://doi.org/10.1111/jcap.12144.

49. Tomoya Hirota et al., "Antiepileptic Medications in Autism Spectrum Disorder: A Systematic Review and Meta-Analysis," *Journal of Autism and Developmental Disorders* 44, no. 4 (2014): 948–57, https://doi.org/10.1007/s10803-013-1952-2.

50. A. Steinbrecher et al., "Supported Decision Making in Delaware," Delaware Network for Excellence in Autism, 2023, https://www.delawareautismnetwork.org/wp-content/uploads/2023/04/SupportedDecision-MakingInDelaware.pdf.

51. Grace I. Hancock, Mark A. Stokes, and Gary B. Mesibov, "Socio-Sexual Functioning in Autism Spectrum Disorder: A Systematic Review and Meta-Analyses of Existing Literature," *Autism Research* 10, no. 11 (2017): 1823–33, https://doi.org/10.1002/aur.1831.

52. "F&D Basic Materials," Friendships and Dating Program, n.d., https://www.fdprogram.org/store/p1/F%26D_Basic_Materials.html.

53. Juliette Bouzy et al., "Transidentities and Autism Spectrum Disorder: A Systematic Review," *Psychiatry Research* 323 (2023): 115176, https://doi.org/10.1016/j.psychres.2023.115176.

CHAPTER 3

1. American Psychiatric Association, *Diagnostic and Statistical Manual of Mental Disorders*, 5th ed., text revision (DSM-5-TR), (Washington, DC: American Psychiatric Association, 2022).

2. Shelly Avenevoli et al., "Major Depression in the National Comorbidity Survey—Adolescent Supplement: Prevalence, Correlates, and Treatment," *Journal of the American Academy of Child & Adolescent Psychiatry* 54, no. 1 (2015): 37–44.

3. A. H. Weinberger et al., "Trends in Depression Prevalence in the USA from 2005 to 2015: Widening Disparities in Vulnerable Groups," *Psychological Medicine* 48, no. 8 (2018): 1308–15, doi: 10.1017/S0033291717002781.

4. "Number and Percentage of Students, by Sexual Identity," Youth Risk Behaviors Surveys, Centers for Disease Control and Prevention, last reviewed April 2023, https://www.cdc.gov/healthyyouth/data/yrbs/supplemental-mmwr/students_by_sexual_identity.htm.

5. "Disparities in Suicide," Suicide Prevention, Centers for Disease Control and Prevention, last modified May 2023, https://www.cdc.gov/suicide/facts/disparities-in-suicide.html.

6. "Youth Risk Behavior Survey Data Summary & Trends Report," Adolescent and School Health, Centers for Disease Control and Prevention, last reviewed April 2023, https://www.cdc.gov/healthyyouth/data/yrbs/pdf/YRBS_Data-Summary-Trends_Report2023_508.pdf.

7. "What Is Self-Injury?," About Self-Injury, International Society for the Study of Self-Injury, last reviewed 2018, https://www.itriples.org/what-is-nssi.

8. Donna Gillies et al., "Prevalence and Characteristics of Self-Harm in Adolescents: Meta-Analyses of Community-Based Studies 1990–2015," *Journal of the American Academy of Child & Adolescent Psychiatry* (October 2018): 737–41, doi: 10.1016/j.jaac.2018.06.018.

9. Keith Hawton et al., "Risk Factors for Suicide in Individuals with Depression: A Systematic Review," *Journal of Affective Disorders* (2013): 17–28, doi: 10.1016/j.jad.2013.01.004.

10. Patrick F. Sullivan, Michael C. Neale, and Kenneth S. Kendler, "Genetic Epidemiology of Major Depression: Review and Meta-Analysis," *American Journal of Psychiatry* 157, no. 10 (2000): 1552–62.

11. Marije aan het Rot, Sanjay J. Mathew, and Dennis S. Charney, "Neurobiological Mechanisms in Major Depressive Disorder," *Canadian Medical Association Journal* 180, no. 3 (2009): 305–13.

12. Kathryn E. Cairns et al., "Risk and Protective Factors for Depression That Adolescents Can Modify: A Systematic Review and Meta-Analysis of Longitudinal Studies," *Journal of Affective Disorders* 169 (2014): 61–75.

13. Jaclyn C. Kearns et al., "Sleep Problems and Suicide Risk in Youth: A Systematic Review, Developmental Framework, and Implications for Hospital Treatment," *General Hospital Psychiatry* 63 (2020): 141–51, https://doi.org/10.1016/j.genhosppsych.2018.09.011.

14. Tamara Chithiramohan and Guy D. Eslick, "Association Between Maternal Postnatal Depression and Offspring Anxiety and Depression in

Adolescence and Young Adulthood: A Meta-Analysis," *Journal of Developmental & Behavioral Pediatrics* 44, no. 3 (2023): e231–e238, https://doi.org/10.1097/DBP.0000000000001164.

15. Danielle Roubinov et al., "Intergenerational Transmission of Maternal Childhood Adversity and Depression on Children's Internalizing Problems," *Journal of Affective Disorders* 308 (2022), 205–12, https://doi.org/10.1016/j.jad.2022.04.030.

16. S. H. Goodman et al., "Parenting as a Mediator of Associations Between Depression in Mothers and Children's Functioning: A Systematic Review and Meta-Analysis," *Clinical Child and Family Psychology Review* (2020), https://doi-org.proxy.library.upenn.edu/10.1007/s10567-020-00322-4.

17. Lyn Y. Abramson, Martin E. Seligman, and John D. Teasdale, "Learned Helplessness in Humans: Critique and Reformulation," *Journal of Abnormal Psychology* 87, no. 1 (1978): 49–74.

18. John R. Z. Abela, Karen Brozina, and Emily P. Haigh, "An Examination of the Response Styles Theory of Depression in Third- and Seventh-Grade Children: A Short-Term Longitudinal Study," *Journal of Abnormal Child Psychology* 30, no. 5 (2002): 515–27.

19. Katrina Witt et al., "Psychosocial Interventions for People Who Self-Harm: Methodological Issues Involved with Trials to Evaluate Effectiveness," *Archives of Suicide Research* (2019), 1–81, doi: 10.1080/13811118.2019.1592043.

20. Jessica Grimmond et al., "A Qualitative Systematic Review of Experiences and Perceptions of Youth Suicide," *PLOS One* (2019), doi: 10.1371/journal.pone.0217569.

21. Di Simes et al., "A Systematic Review of Qualitative Research of the Experiences of Young People and Their Caregivers Affected by Suicidality and Self-Harm: Implications for Family-Based Treatment," *Adolescent Research Review* 7, no. 2: 211–33.

22. Erin C. Dunn et al., "Research Review: Gene-Environment Interaction Research in Youth Depression—A Systematic review with Recommendations for Future Research," *Journal of Child Psychology and Psychiatry* 52, no. 12 (2011): 1223–38.

23. Gianluca Serafini et al., "Life Adversities and Suicidal Behavior in Young Individuals: A Systematic Review," *European Child and Adolescent Psychiatry* (2015), doi: 10.1007/s00787-015-0760-y.

24. Annarosa Cipriano, Stefania Cella, and Paolo Cotrufo, "Nonsuicidal Self-Injury: A Systematic Review," *Frontiers in Psychology* (November 2017), doi: 10.3389/fpsyg.2017.01946.

25. Serafini et al., "Life Adversities and Suicidal Behavior in Young Individuals."

26. Serafini et al., "Life Adversities and Suicidal Behavior in Young Individuals."

27. Simes et al., "Qualitative Research of the Experiences of Young People and Their Caregivers Affected by Suicidality and Self-Harm."

28. Simes et al., "Qualitative Research of the Experiences of Young People and Their Caregivers Affected by Suicidality and Self-Harm."

29. Jonathan M. Platt et al., "Is the US Gender Gap in Depression Changing Over Time? A Meta-Regression," *American Journal of Epidemiology* 190, no. 7, 1190–1206, https://doi.org/10.1093/aje/kwab002.

30. Gillies et al., "Prevalence and Characteristics of Self-Harm in Adolescents."

31. Andrea Miranda-Mendizabal et al., "Gender Differences in Suicidal Behavior in Adolescents and Young Adults: Systematic Review and Meta-Analysis of Longitudinal Studies," *International Journal of Public Health* (March 2019), doi: 10.1007/s00038-018-1196-1.

32. Sherryl H. Goodman and Judy Garber, "Evidence-Based Interventions for Depressed Mothers and Their Young Children," *Child Development Journal* (March 2017), doi: 10.1111/cdev.12732.

33. Ida S. Morken et al., "Explaining the Female Preponderance in Adolescent Depression—A Four-Wave Cohort Study," *Research on Child and Adolescent Psychopathology* 51, no. 6 (2023): 859–69, https://doi.org/10.1007/s10802-023-01031-6.

34. F. Espinosa, N. Martin-Romero, and A. Sanchez-Lopez, "Repetitive Negative Thinking Processes Account for Gender Differences in Depression and Anxiety During Adolescence," *International Journal of Cognitive Therapy* 15, no. 2 (2022), 115–33, https://doi.org/10.1007/s41811-022-00133-1.

35. J. S. Hyde and A. H. Mezulis, "Gender Differences in Depression: Biological, Affective, Cognitive, and Sociocultural Factors," *Harvard Review of Psychiatry* 28, no. 1 (2020): 4–13, https://doi.org/10.1097/HRP.0000000000000230.

36. Pere Castellví et al., "Assessing the Relationship Between School Failure and Suicidal Behavior in Adolescents and Young Adults: A Systematic Review and Meta-Analysis of Longitudinal Studies," *School Mental Health* 12, no. 3 (2020): 429–41, https://doi.org/10.1007/s12310-020-09363-0.

37. Marisa E. Marraccini and Zoe M. F. Brier, "School Connectedness and Suicidal Thoughts and Behaviors: A Systematic Meta-Analysis," *School Psychology Quarterly* (March 2017): 5–21, doi: 10.1037/spq0000192.

38. Lori Shore et al., "Longitudinal Trajectories of Child and Adolescent Depressive Symptoms and Their Predictors–A Systematic Review and Meta-Analysis," *Child and Adolescent Mental Health* 23, no. 2 (2018): 107–20.

39. Ann John et al., "Self-Harm, Suicidal Behaviors, and Cyberbullying in Children and Young People: Systematic Review," *Journal of Medical Internet Research* (2018), doi: 10.2196/jmir.9044.

40. Grimmond et al., "A Qualitative Systematic Review of Experiences and Perceptions of Youth Suicide," *PLOS One* (2019), doi: 10.1371/journal. pone.0217569.

41. Jody Quigley, Susan Rasmussen, and John McAlaney, "The Social Norms of Suicidal and Self-Harming Behaviors in Scottish Adolescents," *International Journal of Environmental Research and Public Health* (2017), http:// dx.doi.ord/10.3390/ijerph14030307.

42. "Youth Risk Behavior Survey Data Summary & Trends Report."

43. Richard T. Liu et al., "Prevalence and Correlates of Non-Suicidal Self-Injury Among Lesbian, Gay, Bisexual, and Transgender Individuals: A Systematic Review and Meta-Analysis," *Clinical Psychology Review* (December 2019), doi: 10.1016/j.cpr.2019.101783.

44. A. Argyriou, K. A. Goldsmith, and K. A. Rimes, "Mediators of the Disparities in Depression Between Sexual Minority and Heterosexual Individuals: A Systematic Review," *Archives of Sexual Behavior* 50, no. 3 (2021), 925–59, https://doi.org/10.1007/s10508-020-01862-0.

45. William Hall, "Psychosocial Risk and Protective Factors for Depression Among Lesbian, Gay, Bisexual, and Queer Youth: A Systematic Review," *Journal of Homosexuality* 65, no. 3 (2018): 263–316, doi: 10.1080/00918369.2017.1317467.

46. Mingli Liu, Lang Wu, and Shuqiao Yao. "Dose–Response Association of Screen Time-Based Sedentary Behaviour in Children and Adolescents and Depression: A Meta-Analysis of Observational Studies," *British Journal of Sports Medicine* 50, no. 20 (2016): 1252–58.

47. Erin Hoare et al., "The Associations Between Sedentary Behaviour and Mental Health Among Adolescents: A Systematic Review," *International Journal of Behavioral Nutrition and Physical Activity*, 13, no. 1 (2016).

48. *Diagnostic and Statistical Manual of Mental Disorders.*

49. Gillies et al., "Prevalence and Characteristics of Self-Harm in Adolescents."

50. Simes et al., "Qualitative Research of the Experiences of Young People and Their Caregivers Affected by Suicidality and Self-Harm."

51. Reem M. Ghandour et al., "Prevalence and Treatment of Depression, Anxiety, and Conduct Problems in US Children," *Journal of Pediatrics* (2020), doi: 10.1016/j.jpeds.2018.09.021.

52. Avenevoli et al., "Major Depression in the National Comorbidity Survey."

53. Greg N. Clarke, P. M. Lewinsohn, and H. Hops, "Adolescent Coping with Depression Course. Kaiser Permanente," *Kaiser Permanente Center for Health Research* (1990), http://www.kpchr.org/acwd/acwd.html.

54. Dikla Eckshtain et al., "Meta-Analysis: 13-Year Follow-Up of Psychotherapy Effects on Youth Depression," *Journal of the American Academy of Child and Adolescent Psychiatry* 59 (2020): 45–63.

55. Sona Dimidjian et al., "The Origins and Current Status of Behavioral Activation Treatments for Depression," *Annual Review of Clinical Psychology* 7 (January 2011): 1–38, https://doi.org/10.1146/annurev-clinpsy-032210-104535.

56. Eckshtain et al., "13-Year Follow-Up of Psychotherapy Effects on Youth Depression."

57. Lucy Tindall et al., "Is Behavioural Activation Effective in the Treatment of Depression in Young People? A Systematic Review and Meta-Analysis," *Psychology and Psychotherapy: Theory, Research, Practice, Training* 90, no. 4 (March 2017): 770–96.

58. Eckshtain et al., "13-Year Follow-Up of Psychotherapy Effects on Youth Depression."

59. Eckshtain et al., "13-Year Follow-Up of Psychotherapy Effects on Youth Depression."

60. Laura H. Mufson et al., *Interpersonal Psychotherapy for Depressed Adolescents*, 2nd ed. (New York: Guilford Press, 2004).

61. J. Liang et al., "Effectiveness Comparisons of Various Psychosocial Therapies for Children and Adolescents with Depression: a Bayesian Network Meta-Analysis," *European Child & Adolescent Psychiatry* 30, no. 5 (2021), 685–97, https://doi.org/10.1007/s00787-020-01492-w.

62. Eckshtain et al., "13-Year Follow-Up of Psychotherapy Effects on Youth Depression."

63. Oswald D. Kothgassner et al., "Efficacy of Dialectical Behavior Therapy for Adolescent Self-Harm and Suicidal Ideation: A Systematic Review and Meta-Analysis," *Psychological Medicine* (2021), doi: 10.1017/S0033291721001355.

64. Lars Mehlum et al., "Dialectical Behavior Therapy for Adolescents with Repeated Suicidal and Self-Harming Behavior: A Randomized Trial," *Journal of the American Academy of Child & Adolescent Psychiatry* (2014): 1082–91, doi: 10.1016/j.jaac.2014.07.003.

65. Marsha M. Linehan, *Cognitive Behavioral Treatment of Borderline Personality Disorder* (New York: Guilford Press, 1993).

66. Colleen Flaherty, "Mental Health Crisis for Grad Students," *Inside Higher Ed* (March 5, 2018).

67. Maya Haasz et al., "Firearms Availability Among High-School Age Youth with Recent Depression or Suicidality," *Pediatrics* 151, no. 6 (2023): 1.

68. J. Elfine, "Percent of Teenagers in the U.S. Taking Antidepressants from 2015 to 2019, by Gender," 2020, https://www.statista.com/statistics/1133612/antidepressant-use-teenagers-by-gender-us/#statisticContainer.

69. Andrea Cipriani et al., "Comparative Efficacy and Tolerability of Antidepressants for Major Depressive Disorder in Children and Adolescents: A Network Meta-Analysis." *The Lancet* (August 2016), doi: 10.1016/S0140-6736(16)30385-3.

70. Sarah E. Hetrick et al., "New Generation Antidepressants for Depression in Children and Adolescents: A Network Meta-Analysis," *Cochrane Library* (May 2021), https://doi.org/10.1002/14651858.CD013674.pub2.

71. Yajie Xiang et al., "Comparative Short-Term Efficacy and Acceptability of a Combination of Pharmacotherapy and Psychotherapy for Depressive Disorder in Children and Adolescents: A Systematic Review and Meta-Analysis," *BMC Psychiatry* 22, no. 1 (February 2022), https://doi.org/10.1186/s12888-022-03760-2.

CHAPTER 4

1. Laiana A. Quagliato, Ursula M. A. de Matos, and Antonio E. Nardi, "Lifetime Psychopathology in the Offspring of Parents with Anxiety Disorders: A Systematic Review," *Journal of Affective Disorders* 319 (2022): 618–26, https://doi.org/10.1016/j.jad.2022.09.049.

2. Olivia Remes et al., "A Systematic Review of Reviews on the Prevalence of Anxiety Disorders in Adult Populations," *Brain and Behavior* 6, no. 7 (2016), https://doi.org/10.1002/brb3.497.

3. Nathan A. Fox et al., "Annual Research Review: Developmental Pathways Linking Early Behavioral Inhibition to Later Anxiety," *Journal of Child Psychology and Psychiatry* 64, no. 4 (2023): 537–61, https://doi.org/10.1111/jcpp.13702.

4. Kirsten Gilbert et al., "Childhood Behavioral Inhibition and Overcontrol: Relationships with Cognitive Functioning, Error Monitoring, Anxiety and Obsessive-Compulsive Symptoms," *Research on Child and Adolescent Psychopathology* 50, no. 12 (2022): 1629–42, https://doi.org/10.1007/s10802-022-00953-x.

5. C. Hong et al., "Global Trends and Regional Differences in the Burden of Anxiety Disorders and Major Depressive Disorder Attributed to Bullying Victimisation in 204 Countries and Territories, 1999–2019: An Analysis of the Global Burden of Disease Study," *Epidemiology and Psychiatric Sciences* 31 (2022): 1999–2009, https://doi.org/10.1017/s2045796022000683.

6. Emily N. Warner et al., "Developmental Epidemiology of Pediatric Anxiety Disorders," *Child and Adolescent Psychiatric Clinics of North America* 32, no. 3 (2023): 511–30, https://doi.org/10.1016/j.chc.2023.02.001.

7. Emily Davey et al., "'It Opened My Eyes': Parents' Experiences of Their Child Receiving an Anxiety Disorder Diagnosis," *Clinical Child Psychology and Psychiatry* 27, no. 3 (2022): 658–69, https://doi.org/10.1177/13591045221088708.

8. Emily N. Warner and Jeffrey R. Strawn, "Risk Factors for Pediatric Anxiety Disorders," *Child and Adolescent Psychiatric Clinics of North America* 32, no. 3 (2023): 485–510, https://doi.org/10.1016/j.chc.2022.10.001.

9. Thomas B. Bertelsen, Joeseph A. Himle, and Åshild Tellefsen Håland, "Bidirectional Relationship Between Family Accommodation and Youth Anxiety During Cognitive-Behavioral Treatment," *Child Psychiatry and Human Development* 54, no. 3 (2023): 905–12, https://doi.org/10.1007/s10578-021-01304-5.

10. Eric A. Storch and Dean McKay, *Obsessive-Compulsive Disorder and Its Spectrum: A Life-Span Approach* (Washington, DC: American Psychological Association, 2014).

11. Joe Kossowsky et al., "The Separation Anxiety Hypothesis of Panic Disorder Revisited: A Meta-Analysis," *American Journal of Psychiatry* 170, no. 7 (2013): 768–81, https://doi.org/10.1176/appi.ajp.2012.12070893.

12. Laura J. Chavez et al., "Trends in Office-Based Anxiety Treatment Among US Children, Youth, and Young Adults: 2006–2018," *Pediatrics* 152, no. 1 (July 2023), e2022059416, 10.1542/peds.2022–059416.

13. Ana Moreno-Alcázar et al., "Efficacy of Eye Movement Desensitization and Reprocessing in Children and Adolescent with Post-Traumatic Stress Disorder: A Meta-Analysis of Randomized Controlled Trials," *Frontiers in Psychology* 8 (2017), https://doi.org/10.3389/fpsyg.2017.01750.

14. Charmaine K. Higa-McMillan et al., "Evidence Base Update: 50 Years of Research on Treatment for Child and Adolescent Anxiety," *Journal of Clinical Child and Adolescent Psychology* 45, no. 2 (2015): 91–113, https://doi.org/10.1080/15374416.2015.1046177.

15. Zoie Wai Tse et al., "School-Based Cognitive-Behavioural Therapy for Children and Adolescents with Social Anxiety Disorder and Social Anxiety Symptoms: A Systematic Review," *PLOS One* 18, no. 3 (2023), https://doi.org/10.1371/journal.pone.0283329.

16. C. Jewell, A. Wittkowski, and D. Pratt, "The Impact of Parent-Only Interventions on Child Anxiety: A Systematic Review and Meta-Analysis," *Journal of Affective Disorders* 309 (2022): 324–49, https://doi.org/10.1016/j.jad.2022.04.082.

17. Anna Lilja Sigurvinsdóttir et al., "Effectiveness of Cognitive Behavioral Therapy (CBT) for Child and Adolescent Anxiety Disorders Across Different CBT Modalities and Comparisons: A Systematic Review and Meta-Analysis," *Nordic Journal of Psychiatry* 74, no. 3 (2019): 168–80, https://doi.org/10.1080/08039488.2019.1686653.

18. Cassandra M. Nicotra and Jeffrey R. Strawn, "Advances in Pharmacotherapy for Pediatric Anxiety Disorders," *Child and Adolescent Psychiatric Clinics of North America* 32, no. 3 (2023): 573–87, https://doi.org/10.1016/j.chc.2023.02.006.

19. Joanna Moncrieff et al., "The Serotonin Theory of Depression: A Systematic Umbrella Review of the Evidence," *Molecular Psychiatry* 28, no. 8 (2022): 3243–56, https://doi.org/10.1038/s41380-022-01661-0.

20. Daniel Wesemann, "Pharmacological Treatment for Pediatric Anxiety Disorders," *Journal of Psychosocial Nursing and Mental Health Services* 60, no. 9 (2022): 6–9, https://doi.org/10.3928/02793695-20220809-04.

21. Sigurvinsdóttir et al., "Effectiveness of Cognitive Behavioral Therapy (CBT) for Child and Adolescent Anxiety Disorders."

22. Yuanmei Tao et al., "Comparing the Efficacy of Pharmacological and Psychological Treatment, Alone and in Combination, in Children and Adolescents with Obsessive-Compulsive Disorder: A Network Meta-Analysis," *Journal of Psychiatric Research* 148 (2022): 95–102, https://doi.org/10.1016/j.jpsychires.2022.01.057.

CHAPTER 5

1. Eric Stice, C. Nathan Marti, and Paul Rohde, "Prevalence, Incidence, Impairment, and Course of the Proposed DSM-5 Eating Disorder Diagnoses in an 8-Year Prospective Community Study of Young Women," *Journal of Abnormal Psychology* 122, no. 2 (2013): 445–57, https://doi.org/10.1037/a0030679.

2. Rachel Bryant-Waugh, "Avoidant/Restrictive Food Intake Disorder," *Child and Adolescent Psychiatric Clinics of North America* 28, no. 4 (2019): 557–65, https://doi.org/10.1016/j.chc.2019.05.004.

3. Jennifer L. Balakar et al., "Recent Advances in Developmental and Risk Factor Research on Eating Disorders," *Current Psychiatry Reports* 17, no. 6 (2015): 1–10, https://doi.org/10.1007/s11920-015-0585-x.

4. Balakar et al., "Developmental and Risk Factor Research."

5. Pernille Stemann Larsen et al., "Parental and Child Characteristics Related to Early-Onset Disordered Eating," *Harvard Review of Psychiatry* 18, no. 3 (2015): 183–202, https://doi.org/10.1097/hrp.0000000000000073.

6. Balakar et al., "Developmental and Risk Factor Research."

7. Lisa R. R. Lilenfeld et al., "Eating Disorders and Personality: A Methodological and Empirical Review," *Clinical Psychology Review* 26, no. 3 (2006): 299–320, https://doi.org/10.1016/j.cpr.2005.10.003.

8. Balakar et al., "Developmental and Risk Factor Research."

9. Ziporah B. Henderson et al., "Emotional Development in Eating Disorders: A Qualitative Metasynthesis," *Clinical Psychology & Psychotherapy* 26, no. 4 (2019): 440–57, https://doi.org/10.1002/cpp.2365.

10. Balakar et al., "Developmental and Risk Factor Research."

11. Eng Joo Tan et al., "The Association Between Eating Disorders and Mental Health: An Umbrella Review," *Journal of Eating Disorders* 11, no. 1 (2023), https://doi.org/10.1186/s40337-022-00725-4.

12. Marco Solmi et al., "Age at Onset of Mental Disorders Worldwide: Large-Scale Meta-Analysis of 192 Epidemiological Studies," *Molecular Psychiatry* 27 (2022): 281–95, https://doi.org/10.1038/s41380-021-01161-7.

13. Alexandra Dane and Komal Bhatia, "The Social Media Diet: A Scoping Review to Investigate the Association Between Social Media, Body Image and Eating Disorders Amongst Young People," *PLOS Global Public Health* 3, no. 3 (2023), https://doi.org/10.1371/journal.pgph.0001091.

14. Jorunn Sundgot-Borgen and Monica Klungland Torstveit, "Prevalence of Eating Disorders in Elite Athletes Is Higher Than in the General Population," *Clinical Journal of Sport Medicine* 14, no. 1 (2004): 25–32, https://doi.org/10.1097/00042752-200401000-00005.

15. Anna Riva et al., "Eating Disorders in Children and Adolescent Males: A Peculiar Psychopathological Profile," *International Journal of Environmental Research and Public Health* 19, no. 18 (2022): 11449, https://doi.org/10.3390/ijerph191811449.

16. Sonja A. Swanson et al., "Prevalence and Correlates of Eating Disorders in Adolescents," *Archives of General Psychiatry* 68, no. 7 (2011): 714, https://doi.org/10.1001/archgenpsychiatry.2011.22.

17. Balakar et al., "Developmental and Risk Factor Research."

18. James Lock and Maria C. La Via, "Practice Parameter for the Assessment and Treatment of Children and Adolescents with Eating Disorders," *Journal of the American Academy of Child & Adolescent Psychiatry* 54, no. 5 (2015): 412–25, https://doi.org/10.1016/j.jaac.2015.01.018.

19. Lock and La Via, "Assessment and Treatment."

20. Caterina Filipponi et al., "The Follow-Up of Eating Disorders from Adolescence to Early Adulthood: A Systematic Review," *International Journal of Environmental Research and Public Health* 19, no. 23 (2022): 16237, https://doi.org/10.3390/ijerph192316237.

21. Lock and La Via, "Assessment and Treatment."

22. Lock and La Via, "Assessment and Treatment."

23. James Lock, "Updates on Treatments for Adolescent Anorexia Nervosa," *Child and Adolescent Psychiatric Clinics of North America* 28, no. 4 (2019): 523–35, https://doi.org/10.1016/j.chc.2019.05.001.

24. Joel Yager et al., "Guideline Watch (August 2012): Practice Guideline for the Treatment of Patients with Eating Disorders, 3rd Edition," *FOCUS* 12, no. 4 (2014): 416–31, https://doi.org/10.1176/appi.focus.120404.

25. Tiffany A. Graves et al., "A Meta-Analysis of the Relation Between Therapeutic Alliance and Treatment Outcome in Eating Disorders," *International Journal of Eating Disorders* 50, no. 4 (2017): 323–40, https://doi.org/10.1002/eat.22672.

26. Lock and La Via, "Assessment and Treatment."

27. Keren Friedman et al., "A Narrative Review of Outcome Studies for Residential and Partial Hospital-Based Treatment of Eating Disorders," *Journal of the Eating Disorders Association* 24, no. 4 (2016): 263–76, https://doi.org/10.1002/erv.2449.

28. N. Golden et al., "Position Paper of the Society for Adolescent Health and Medicine: Medical Management of Restrictive Eating Disorders in Adolescents and Young Adults," *Journal of Adolescent Health* 56, no. 1 (2015): 121–25.

29. James Lock and Daniel Le Grange, "Family□Based Treatment: Where Are We and Where Should We Be Going to Improve Recovery in Child and Adolescent Eating Disorders," *International Journal of Eating Disorders* 52, no. 4 (2018): 481–87, https://doi.org/10.1002/eat.22980.

30. Lock and Le Grange, "Family-Based Treatment."

31. Daniel Le Grange et al., "Randomized Clinical Trial of Family-Based Treatment and Cognitive-Behavioral Therapy for Adolescent Bulimia Nervosa," *Journal of the American Academy of Child & Adolescent Psychiatry* 54, no. 11 (2015): 886–94, https://doi.org/10.1016/j.jaac.2015.08.008.

32. Lock and Le Grange, "Family-Based Treatment."

33. Nandini Datta et al., "Evidence Based Update on Psychosocial Treatments for Eating Disorders in Children and Adolescents," *Official Journal for the Society of Clinical Child and Adolescent Psychology, American Psychological Association* 52, no. 2 (2023): 159–70, https://doi.org/10.1080/15374416.2022.2109650.

34. Datta et al., "Psychosocial Treatments for Eating Disorders."

35. Riccardo Dalle Grave, Massimiliano Sartirana, and Simona Calugi, "Enhanced Cognitive Behavioral Therapy for Adolescents with Anorexia Nervosa: Outcomes and Predictors of Change in a Real-World Setting," *International Journal of Eating Disorders* 52, no. 9 (2019): 1042–46, https://doi.org/10.1002/eat.23122.

36. David M. Garner et al., "Psychotropic Medications in Adult and Adolescent Eating Disorders: Clinical Practice versus Evidence-Based Recommendations," *Eating and Weight Disorders—Studies on Anorexia, Bulimia and Obesity* 21, no. 3 (2016): 395–402, https://doi.org/10.1007/s40519-016-0253-0.

37. Lock and La Via, "Assessment and Treatment."

38. Jennifer Couturier et al., "Psychotropic Medication for Children and Adolescents with Eating Disorders," *Child and Adolescent Psychiatric Clinics of North America* 28, no. 4 (2019): 583–92, https://doi.org/10.1016/j.chc.2019.05.005.

39. Lock, "Treatments for Adolescent Anorexia Nervosa."

CHAPTER 6

1. American Psychiatric Association, *Diagnostic and Statistical Manual,* 5th ed., text revision (DSM-5-TR) (Washington, DC: American Psychiatric Association, 2022).

2. Viktoria Vibkufar et al., "A Systematic Review and Meta-Analysis on the Prevalence of Depression in Children and Adolescents After Exposure to Trauma," *Journal of Affective Disorders* 255 (2019): 77–89, https://doi.org/doi.org/10.1016/j.jad.2019.05.005.

3. Jeffrey Guina et al. "Should Posttraumatic Stress Be a Disorder or a Specifier?" *Current Psychiatry Reports* 19 (2017), https://doi.org/10.1007/s11920-017-0821-7.

4. World Health Organization, *International Classification of Disorders,* 11th revision, https://www.who.int/standards/classifications/classification-of-diseases.

5. Katie McLaughlin et al., "Trauma Exposure and Posttraumatic Stress Disorder in a National Sample of Adolescents," *Journal of the American Academy of Child & Adolescent Psychiatry* 52, no. 8 (2013): 815–30, https://doi.org/doi.org/10.1016/j.jaac.2013.05.011.

6. Francesca Woolgar et al., "Systematic Review and Meta-Analysis: Prevalence of Posttraumatic Stress Disorder in Trauma-Exposed Preschool-Aged Children," *Journal of the American Academy of Child and Adolescent Psychiatry* 61, no. 3 (2022): 366–77, https://doi.org/doi.org/10.1016/j.jaac.2021.05.026.

7. Eva Alisic et al., "Rates of Post-Traumatic Stress Disorder in Trauma-Exposed Children and Adolescents: Meta-Analysis," *British Journal of Psychiatry* 204, no. 5 (2014): 335–40, https://doi.org/10.1192/bjp.bp.113.131227.

8. McLaughlin et al., "Trauma Exposure and Posttraumatic Stress."

9. Jessica Memarzia, Jack Walker, and Richard Meiser-Stedman, "Psychological Peritraumatic Risk Factors for Post-Traumatic Stress Disorder in Children and Adolescents: A Meta-Analytic Review," *Journal of Affective Disorders* 282 (2021): 1036–47, https://doi.org/10.1016/j.jad.2021.01.016.

10. Aaron Levin, "Early Life Trauma Changes Biology of Brain," *Psychiatric News* 54, no. 14 (2019), https://doi.org/10.1176/appi.pn.2019.6b19.

11. Pingxing Xie et al., "Interactive Effect of Stressful Life Events and the Serotonin Transporter 5-HTTLPR Genotype on Posttraumatic Stress Disorder Diagnosis in 2 Independent Populations," *Archives of General Psychiatry* 66, no. 11 (2009): 1201, https://doi.org/10.1001/archgenpsychiatry.2009.153.

12. Judith A. Cohen, Esther Deblinger, and Anthony P. Mannarino, *Treating Trauma and Traumatic Grief in Children and Adolescents*, 2nd ed. (New York: Guilford Press, 2017).

13. Leila Allen et al., "The Correlation Between Social Support and Post-Traumatic Stress Disorder in Children and Adolescents: A Meta-Analysis," *Journal of Affective Disorders* 294 (2021): 543–57, https://doi.org/10.1016/j.jad.2021.07.028.

14. Woolgar et al., "Prevalence of Posttraumatic Stress Disorder in Trauma-Exposed Preschool-Aged Children."

15. McLaughlin et al., "Trauma Exposure and Posttraumatic Stress."

16. Raphaël Arditti and Yann Le Strat, "A Traumatic Life Experience in Childhood Increases the Risk of a Psychiatric Disorder in the Offspring," *Psychiatry Research* 290 (2020): 113101, https://doi.org/10.1016/j.psychres.2020.113101.

17. Rachel M. Hiller et al., "A Longitudinal Investigation of the Role of Parental Responses in Predicting Children's Post-Traumatic Distress," *Journal of Child Psychology and Psychiatry* 59, no. 7 (2018): 781–89, https://doi.org/10.1111/jcpp.12846.

18. Nexhmedin Morina, Rachel Koerssen, and Thomas V. Pollet, "Interventions for Children and Adolescents with Posttraumatic Stress Disorder: A Meta-Analysis of Comparative Outcome Studies," *Clinical Psychology Review* 47 (2016): 41–54, https://doi.org/10.1016/j.cpr.2016.05.006.

19. Chen-Yang Xian-Yu et al. "Cognitive Behavioral Therapy for Children and Adolescents with Post-Traumatic Stress Disorder: Meta-Analysis," *Journal of Affective Disorders* 308 (2022): 502–11, doi:10.1016/j.jad.2022.04.111.

20. Phyllis Lee and Jason M. Lang, "Comparing Trauma-Focused Cognitive-Behavioral Therapy to Commonly Used Treatments in Usual Care for Children with Posttraumatic Stress Disorder," *Psychological Trauma: Theory, Research, Practice, and Policy*, 2023, https://doi.org/10.1037/tra0001555.

21. Christina Gamache Martin et al., "The Role of Caregiver Psychopathology in the Treatment of Childhood Trauma with Trauma-Focused Cognitive Behavioral Therapy: A Systematic Review," *Clinical Child and Family Psychology Review* 22, no. 3 (2019): 273–89, https://doi.org/10.1007/s10567-019-00290-4.

22. Jaxon J. Humble et al., "Child-Centered Play Therapy for Youths Who Have Experienced Trauma: A Systematic Literature Review," *Journal of Child*

& Adolescent Trauma 12, no. 3 (2018): 365–75, https://doi.org/10.1007/s40653 -018-0235-7.

23. Dee C. Ray, *Advanced Play Therapy: Essential Conditions, Knowledge, and Skills for Child Practice* (New York: Routledge, Taylor & Francis Group, 2021).

24. Mark C. Russell and Francine Shapiro, *Eye Movement Desensitization and Reprocessing (EMDR) Therapy* (Washington, DC: American Psychological Association, 2022).

25. Patricia Novo Navarro et al., "25 Años de Eye Movement Desensitization and Reprocessing: Protocolo de Aplicación, Hipótesis de Funcionamiento y Revisión Sistemática de Su Eficacia En El Trastorno Por Estrés Postraumático," *Revista de Psiquiatría y Salud Mental* 11, no. 2 (2018): 101–14, https://doi.org/10.1016/j.rpsm.2015.12.002.

26. Ana Moreno-Alcázar et al. "Efficacy of Eye Movement Desensitization and Reprocessing in Children and Adolescent with Post-Traumatic Stress Disorder: A Meta-Analysis of Randomized Controlled Trials." *Frontiers in Psychology* 8 (2017), doi.10.3389/fpsyg.2017.01750.

27. Rene Soria-Saucedo et al., "Factors That Predict the Use of Psychotropics Among Children and Adolescents with PTSD: Evidence from Private Insurance Claims," *Psychiatric Services* 69, no. 9 (2018): 1007–14, https://doi .org/10.1176/appi.ps.201700167.

28. *Diagnostic and Statistical Manual.*

29. *Diagnostic and Statistical Manual.*

30. https://childparentpsychotherapy.com.

31. https://www.connectattachmentprograms.org.

32. *Diagnostic and Statistical Manual.*

CHAPTER 7

1. American Psychiatric Association, *Diagnostic and Statistical Manual of Mental Disorders* (DSM-5-TR) (Washington, DC: American Psychiatric Association, 2022).

2. Helen Link Egger and Adrian Angold, "Common Emotional and Behavioral Disorders in Preschool Children: Presentation, Nosology, and Epidemiology," *Journal of Child Psychology and Psychiatry* 47, no. 3–4 (2006): 313–37, https://doi.org/10.1111/j.1469-7610.2006.01618.x.

3. Ellen M. Kessel et al., "Early Predictors of Adolescent Irritability," *Child and Adolescent Psychiatric Clinics of North America* 30, no. 3 (2021): 475–90, https://doi.org/10.1016/j.chc.2021.04.002.

4. Daniel N. Klein et al., "A Transdiagnostic Perspective on Youth Irritability," *Current Directions in Psychological Science* 30, no. 5 (2021): 437–43, https://doi.org/10.1177/09637214211035101.

5. *Diagnostic Manual of Mental Disorders.*

6. Qiongru Yu et al., "Roads Diverged: Developmental Trajectories of Irritability from Toddlerhood through Adolescence," *Journal of the American Academy of Child and Adolescent Psychiatry* 62, no. 4 (2023): 457–71, https://doi.org/10.1016/j.jaac.2022.07.849.

7. Brian M. Hicks et al., "Environmental Adversity and Increasing Genetic Risk for Externalizing Disorders," *Archives of General Psychiatry* 66, no. 6 (2009): 640–48, https://doi.org/10.1001/archgenpsychiatry.2008.554.

8. J. Nigg and C. Huang-Pollock, "An Early-Onset Model of the Role of Executive Functions and Intelligence in Conduct Disorder/Delinquency," in B. Lahey, T. E. Moffitt, & A. Caspi (eds.), *Causes of Conduct Disorder and Juvenile Delinquency* (New York: Guilford Press, 2003), 227–53.

9. Getinet Ayano et al., "The Risk of Anxiety Disorders in Children of Parents with Severe Psychiatric Disorders: A Systematic Review and Meta-Analysis," *Journal of Affective Disorders* 282 (2021): 472–87, https://doi.org/10.1016/j.jad.2020.12.134.

10. Berihun Assefa Dachew et al., "Association of Maternal Depressive Symptoms During the Perinatal Period with Oppositional Defiant Disorder in Children and Adolescents," *JAMA Network Open* 4, no. 9 (2021), https://doi.org/10.1001/jamanetworkopen.2021.25854.

11. Joel Stoddard et al., "An Open Pilot Study of Training Hostile Interpretation Bias to Treat Disruptive Mood Dysregulation Disorder," *Journal of Child and Adolescent Psychopharmacology* 26, no. 1 (2016): 49–57, https://doi.org/10.1089/cap.2015.0100.

12. Stephanie G. Craig et al., "The Mediational Effect of Affect Dysregulation on the Association between Attachment to Parents and Oppositional Defiant Disorder Symptoms in Adolescents," *Child Psychiatry and Human Development* 52, no. 5 (2020): 818–28, https://doi.org/10.1007/s10578-020-01059-5.

13. Raúl Navarro et al., "Families, Parenting and Aggressive Preschoolers: A Scoping Review of Studies Examining Family Variables Related to Preschool Aggression," *International Journal of Environmental Research and Public Health* 19, no. 23 (2022): 15556, https://doi.org/10.3390/ijerph192315556.

14. Xiuyun Lin et al., "A Systematic Review of Multiple Family Factors Associated with Oppositional Defiant Disorder," *International Journal of Environmental Research and Public Health* 19, no. 17 (2022): 10866, https://doi.org/10.3390/ijerph191710866.

15. Foster Cline and Jim Fay, *Parenting with Love and Logic: Teaching Children Responsibility* (Carol Stream, IL: NavPress Publishing Group, 2020).

16. "Child Maltreatment 2019: Summary of Key Findings," Child Welfare Information Gateway, n.d., https://www.childwelfare.gov/pubs/factsheets /canstats/.

17. Oliver Perra, Amy L. Paine, and Dale F. Hay, "Continuity and Change in Anger and Aggressiveness from Infancy to Childhood: The Protective Effects of Positive Parenting," *Development and Psychopathology* 33, no. 3 (2020): 937–56, https://doi.org/10.1017/s0954579420000243.

18. Lauren Markham, *Peaceful Parent, Happy Kids: How to Stop Yelling and Start Connecting* (New York: Perigee Book, 2012).

19. Hicks et al., "Risk for Externalizing Disorders," 640–48.

20. Alan E. Kazdin, *The Kazdin Method for Parenting the Defiant Child: With No Pills, No Therapy, No Contest of Wills* (Harper, 2009).

21. Kazdin, *Parenting the Defiant Child.*

22. R. C. Berg, et al., *Interventions for Children and Youth with Behavioural Problems or Criminal Behaviour: An Overview of Reviews.* Norwegian Institute of Public Health, 2020.

23. Markham, *Peaceful Parent, Happy Kids.*

24. John E. Lochman et al., "Cognitive-Behavioral Therapy for Externalizing Disorders in Children and Adolescents," *Child and Adolescent Psychiatric Clinics of North America* 20, no. 2 (2011): 305–18, https://doi.org/10.1016/j .chc.2011.01.005.

25. Ji-Woo Seok et al., "Psychopharmacological Treatment of Disruptive Behavior in Youths: Systematic Review and Network Meta-Analysis," *Scientific Reports* 13, no. 1 (2023), https://doi.org/10.1038/s41598-023-33979-2.

26. Drew E. Winters et al., "Improvements in Irritability with Open-Label Methylphenidate Treatment in Youth with Comorbid Attention Deficit/Hyperactivity Disorder and Disruptive Mood Dysregulation Disorder," *Journal of Child and Adolescent Psychopharmacology* 28, no. 5 (2018): 298–305, https:// doi.org/10.1089/cap.2017.0124.

27. Jik H. Loy et al., "Atypical Antipsychotics for Disruptive Behaviour Disorders in Children and Youths," *Cochrane Database of Systematic Reviews* 2017, no. 8 (2017), https://doi.org/10.1002/14651858.cd008559.pub3.

CHAPTER 8

1. Seongju Kim and Dohyung Kim, "Behavioral Symptoms of Child Mental Disorders and Lifetime Substance Use in Adolescence: A Within-Family Comparison of US Siblings," *Drug and Alcohol Dependence* 219 (2021): 108490, https://doi.org/10.1016/j.drugalcdep.2020.108490.

2. American Psychiatric Association, *Diagnostic and Statistical Manual of Mental Disorders* (DSM-5-TR) (Washington, DC: American Psychiatric Association, 2022).

3. Richard Rowe et al., "Developmental Pathways in Oppositional Defiant Disorder and Conduct Disorder," *Journal of Abnormal Psychology* 119, no. 4 (2010): 726–38, https://doi.org/10.1037/a0020798.

4. J. Friedman et al., "Trends in Drug Overdose Deaths Among US Adolescents, January 2010 to June 2021, *JAMA* 327, no. 14 (2022): 1398–1400, doi:10.1001/jama.2022.2847.

5. Youth Risk Behavior Survey—Centers for Disease Control and Prevention, n.d., https://www.cdc.gov/healthyyouth/data/yrbs/pdf/YRBS_Data-Summary-Trends_Report2023_508.pdf?mc_cid=d112968ed9&mc_eid=80b51934b7.

6. C. C. W. Lim et al., Prevalence of Adolescent Cannabis Vaping: A Systematic Review and Meta-Analysis of US and Canadian Studies, *JAMA Pediatrics* 176, no. 1 (2022): 42–51, doi:10.1001/jamapediatrics.2021.4102.

7. Christian J. Hopper, Thomas J. Crowley, and John K. Hewitt, "Review of Twin and Adoption Studies of Adolescent Substance Use," *Journal of the American Academy of Child & Adolescent Psychiatry* 42, no. 6 (2003): 710–19, https://doi.org/10.1097/01.chi.0000046848.56865.54.

8. S. G. Craig, N. Goulter, and M. M. Moretti, "A Systematic Review of Primary and Secondary Callous-Unemotional Traits and Psychopathy Variants in Youth," *Clinical Child and Family Psychology Review* 24, no. 1 (2021): 65–91, https://doi.org/10.1007/s10567-020-00329-x.

9. Rene Carbonneau et al., "Early Risk Factors Associated with Preschool Developmental Patterns of Single and Co-Occurrent Disruptive Behaviors in a Population Sample," *Developmental Psychology* 58, no. 3 (2022): 438–52, https://doi.org/10.1037/dev0001295.

10. Carlos Andres Trujillo, Diana Obando, and Angela Trujillo, "An Examination of the Association between Early Initiation of Substance Use and Interrelated Multilevel Risk and Protective Factors Among Adolescents," *PLOS One* 14, no. 12 (2019), https://doi.org/10.1371/journal.pone.0225384.

11. Brian T. Wymbs et al., "Early Adolescent Substance Use as a Risk Factor for Developing Conduct Disorder and Depression Symptoms," *Journal of Studies on Alcohol and Drugs* 75, no. 2 (2014): 279–89, https://doi.org/10.15288/jsad.2014.75.279.

12. Azmawati Mohammed Nawi et al., "Risk and Protective Factors of Drug Abuse Among Adolescents: A Systematic Review," *BMC Public Health* 21, no. 1 (2021), https://doi.org/10.1186/s12889-021-11906-2.

13. Aaron Hogue et al., "Evidence Base on Outpatient Behavioral Treatments for Adolescent Substance Use: Updates and Recommendations 2007–2013," *Journal of Clinical Child & Adolescent Psychology* 43, no. 5 (2018): 695–720, https://doi.org/10.1080/15374416.2014.915550.

14. Angelica M. Morales et al., "Identifying Early Risk Factors for Addiction Later in Life: A Review of Prospective Longitudinal Studies," *Current Addiction Reports* 7, no. 1 (2019): 89–98, https://doi.org/10.1007/s40429-019 -00282-y.

15. Timothy E. Wilens et al., "The Impact of Pharmacotherapy of Childhood-Onset Psychiatric Disorders on the Development of Substance Use Disorders," *Journal of Child and Adolescent Psychopharmacology* 32, no. 4 (2022): 200–14, https://doi.org/10.1089/cap.2022.0016.

16. Nawi et al., "Risk and Protective Factors."

17. Craig, Goulter, and Moretti, "Primary and Secondary Callous-Unemotional Traits."

18. Abigail A. Fagan, "Child Maltreatment and Aggressive Behaviors in Early Adolescence: Evidence of Moderation by Parent/Child Relationship Quality," *Child Maltreatment* 25, no. 2 (2019): 182–91, https://doi.org/10.1177 /1077559519874401.

19. Lindsay A. Taliaferro et al., "Profiles of Risk and Protection for Violence and Bullying Perpetration Among Adolescent Boys," *Journal of School Health* 90, no. 3 (2020): 212–23, https://doi.org/10.1111/josh.12867.

20. Taliaferro et al., "Violence and Bullying Perpetration among Adolescent Boys."

21. Carbonneau et al., "Early Risk Factors Associated with Preschool Developmental Patterns."

22. Vincent Bégin et al., "Perinatal and Early-Life Factors Associated with Stable and Unstable Trajectories of Psychopathic Traits Across Childhood," *Psychological Medicine* 53, no. 2 (2023): 379–87, https://doi.org/10.1017/ s0033291721001586.

23. Ellen M. Kessel et al., "Early Predictors of Adolescent Irritability," *Child and Adolescent Psychiatric Clinics of North America* 30, no. 3 (2021): 475–90, https://doi.org/10.1016/j.chc.2021.04.002.

24. Monika A. Waszczuk, Helena M. Zavos, and Thalia C. Eley, "Why Do Depression, Conduct, and Hyperactivity Symptoms Co-Occur Across Adolescence? The Role of Stable and Dynamic Genetic and Environmental Influences," *European Child & Adolescent Psychiatry* 30, no. 7 (2021): 1013–25, https://doi.org/10.1007/s00787-020-01515-6.

25. Emily J. LoBraico et al., "Constellations of Family Risk for Long-Term Adolescent Antisocial Behavior," *Journal of Family Psychology* 34, no. 5 (2020): 587–97, https://doi.org/10.1037/fam0000640.

26. Carbonneau et al., "Early Risk Factors Associated with Preschool Developmental Patterns."

27. Carbonneau et al., "Early Risk Factors Associated with Preschool Developmental Patterns."

28. Allegra S. Anderson et al., "Parental Drug Use Disorders and Youth Psychopathology: Meta-Analytic Review," *Drug and Alcohol Dependence* 244 (2023): 109793, https://doi.org/10.1016/j.drugalcdep.2023.109793.

29. Kessel et al., "Early Predictors of Adolescent Irritability."

30. Hogue et al., "Outpatient Behavioral Treatments."

31. Angela K. Henneberger, Dawnsha R. Mushonga, and Alison M. Preston, "Peer Influence and Adolescent Substance Use: A Systematic Review of Dynamic Social Network Research," *Adolescent Research Review* 6, no. 1 (2021): 57–73, https://doi.org/10.1007/s40894-019-00130-0.

32. Matthew C. Fadus et al., "Unconscious Bias and the Diagnosis of Disruptive Behavior Disorders and ADHD in African American and Hispanic Youth," *Academic Psychiatry* 44, no. 1 (2020): 95–102, https://doi.org/10.1007/s40596 -019-01127-6.

33. Carbonneau et al., "Early Risk Factors Associated with Preschool Developmental Patterns."

34. Kessel et al., "Early Predictors of Adolescent Irritability."

35. Patricia Logan-Greene et al., "Protective Factors Against Aggression and Antisocial Attitudes Among Probation Youth with Childhood Adversity Histories," *Prevention Science* 24, no. 1 (2022): 161–72, https://doi.org/10.1007/ s11121-022-01472-3.

36. Azmawati Mohammed Nawi et al., "Risk and Protective Factors of Drug Abuse Among Adolescents: A Systematic Review," *BMC Public Health* 21, no. 1 (2021), https://doi.org/10.1186/s12889-021-11906-2.

37. Alexis Yohros, "Examining the Relationship Between Adverse Childhood Experiences and Juvenile Recidivism: A Systematic Review and Meta-Analysis," *Trauma, Violence, & Abuse* 24, no. 3 (2023): 1640–55, https: //doi.org/10.1177/15248380211073846.

38. Michael T. Baglivio et al., "The Role of Adverse Childhood Experiences (Aces) and Psychopathic Features on Juvenile Offending Criminal Careers to Age 18," *Youth Violence and Juvenile Justice* 18, no. 4 (2020): 337–64, https: //doi.org/10.1177/1541204020927075.

39. Nawi et al., "Risk and Protective Factors of Drug Abuse Among Adolescents."

40. Aaron L. Sarvet et al., "Medical Marijuana Laws and Adolescent Marijuana Use in the United States: A Systematic Review and Meta-Analysis," *Addiction* 113, no. 6 (2018): 1003–16, https://doi.org/10.1111/add.14136.

41. Yuyan Shi, Sharon E. Cummins, and Shu-Hong Zhu, "Medical Marijuana Availability, Price, and Product Variety, and Adolescents' Marijuana Use," *Journal of Adolescent Health* 63, no. 1 (2018): 88–93, https://doi.org/10.1016 /j.jadohealth.2018.01.008.

42. Rebekah Levine Coley et al., "A Quasi-Experimental Evaluation of Marijuana Policies and Youth Marijuana Use," *American Journal of Drug and*

Alcohol Abuse 45, no. 3 (2019): 292–303, https://doi.org/10.1080/00952990.2018.1559847.

43. Kayla N. Tormohlen et al., "Changes in Prevalence of Marijuana Consumption Modes Among Colorado High School Students from 2015 to 2017," *JAMA Pediatrics* 173, no. 10 (2019): 988–89, https://doi.org/10.1001/jamapediatrics.2019.2627.

44. Mary Frances Mullins, "Cannabis Dabbing," *Nursing* 51, no. 5 (2021): 46–50, https://doi.org/10.1097/01.nurse.0000743108.72528.d8.

45. Hogue et al., "Outpatient Behavioral Treatments."

46. Steve Sussman, "A Review of Alcoholics Anonymous / Narcotics Anonymous Programs for Teens," *Evaluation & the Health Professions* 33, no. 1 (2010): 26–55, https://doi.org/10.1177/.

47. Aaron Hogue et al., "Core Elements of CBT for Adolescent Conduct and Substance Use Problems: Comorbidity, Clinical Techniques, and Case Examples," *Cognitive and Behavioral Practice* 27, no. 4 (2020): 426–41, https://doi.org/10.1016/j.cbpra.2019.12.002.

48. Emily E. Tanner-Smith, Sandra Jo Wilson, and Mark W. Lipsey, "The Comparative Effectiveness of Outpatient Treatment for Adolescent Substance Abuse: A Meta-Analysis," *Journal of Substance Abuse Treatment* 44, no. 2 (2013): 145–58, https://doi.org/10.1016/j.jsat.2012.05.006.

49. Alex R. Dopp et al., "Family-Based Treatments for Serious Juvenile Offenders: A Multilevel Meta-Analysis," *Journal of Consulting and Clinical Psychology* 85, no. 4 (2017): 335–54.

50. Brad Donohue et al., "Family Behavior Therapy for Substance Abuse and Other Associated Problems," *Behavior Modification* 33, no. 5 (2009): 495–519, https://doi.org/10.1177/0145445509340019.

51. P. Chamberlain and D. K. Smith, "Antisocial Behavior in Children and Adolescents: The Oregon Multidimensional Treatment Foster Care Model," in A. E. Kazdin and J. R. Weisz (eds.), Evidence-Based Psychotherapies for Children and Adolescents (New York: Guilford Press, 2003), 282–300.

52. James Alexander and Bruce V. Parsons, *Functional Family Therapy* (Monterey, CA: Brooks/Cole, 1982).

53. Howard A. Liddle et al., "Multidimensional Family Therapy for Adolescent Drug Abuse: Results of a Randomized Clinical Trial," *American Journal of Drug and Alcohol Abuse* 27, no. 4 (2001): 651–88, https://doi.org/10.1081/ada-100107661.

54. S. W. Henggeler et al., "Effects of Multisystemic Therapy on Drug Use and Abuse in Serious Juvenile Offenders: A Progress Report from Two Outcome Studies," Family Dynamics of Addiction Quarterly 1, no. 3 (1991): 40–51.

55. Cindy M. Schaeffer et al., "A Smartphone App for Parental Management of Adolescent Conduct Problems: Randomized Clinical Trial of iKinnect," *Journal of Clinical Child and Adolescent Psychology* (2022): 1–15.

56. Seena Fazel, Helen Doll, and Niklas Langstrom, "Mental Disorders Among Adolescents in Juvenile Detention and Correctional Facilities: A Systematic Review and Metaregression Analysis of 25 Surveys," *Journal of the American Academy of Child and Adolescent Psychiatry* 47, no. 9 (2008): 1010–19.

57. Chye Toole-Anstey, Lynne Keevers, and Michelle L. Townsend, "A Systematic Review of Child to Parent Violence Interventions," *Trauma, Violence, & Abuse* 24, no. 2 (2023): 1157–71, https://doi.org/10.1177/15248380211053618.

58. Child to Parent Violence (CPV)—proceduresonline.com, accessed June 24, 2023, https://proceduresonline.com/nesubregion/files/southtyne_cpv.pdf.

59. Robert Miranda and Hayley Treloar, "Emerging Pharmacologic Treatments for Adolescent Substance Use: Challenges and New Directions," *Current Addiction Reports* 3, no. 2 (2016): 145–56, https://doi.org/10.1007/s40429-016-0098-7.

60. Jessica L. Hambly et al., "Pharmacotherapy of Conduct Disorder: Challenges, Options and Future Directions," *Journal of Psychopharmacology* 30, no. 10 (2016): 967–75, https://doi.org/10.1177/0269881116658985.

61. Jik H. Loy et al., "Atypical Antipsychotics for Disruptive Behaviour Disorders in Children and Youths," *Cochrane Database of Systematic Reviews* 2017, no. 8 (2017), https://doi.org/10.1002/14651858.cd008559.pub3.

62. Hambly et al., "Pharmacotherapy of Conduct Disorder."

CHAPTER 9

1. Shabnam Javdani, McKenzie N. Berezin, and Keisha April, "A Treatment-to-Prison-Pipeline? Scoping Review and Multimethod Examination of Legal Consequences of Residential Treatment Among Adolescents," *Journal of Clinical Child & Adolescent Psychology* 52, no. 3 (2023): 376–95, https://doi.org/10.1080/15374416.2023.2178003.

2. Joanna E. Bettmann et al., "A Meta-Analysis of Wilderness Therapy Outcomes for Private Pay Clients," *Journal of Child and Family Studies* 25, no. 9 (2016): 2659–73, https://doi.org/10.1007/s10826-016-0439-0.

3. Natalie Beck and Jennifer S. Wong, "A Meta-Analysis of the Effects of Wilderness Therapy on Delinquent Behaviors Among Youth," *Criminal Justice and Behavior Criminal Justice and Behavior* 49, no. 5 (2022): 700–729, https://doi.org/10.21428/cb6ab371.e81872f8.

4. J. Cramer and P. Wanner, "Wilderness Therapy Programs: A Systematic Review of Research," June 2022, https://www.wsipp.wa.gov/ReportFile/1748 /Wsipp_Wilderness-Therapy-Programs-A-Systematic-Review-of-Research _Report.pdf.

5. Frederic G. Reamer and Deborah H. Siegel, *Teens in Crisis: How the Industry Serving Struggling Teens Helps and Hurts Our Kids* (New York: Columbia University Press, 2008).

6. Sarah Golightley, "Troubling the 'Troubled Teen' Industry: Adult Reflections on Youth Experiences of Therapeutic Boarding Schools," *Global Studies of Childhood* 10, no. 1 (2020): 53–63, https://doi.org/10.1177 /2043610619900514.

7. Lenore Behar et al., "Protecting Youth Placed in Unlicensed, Unregulated Residential 'Treatment' Facilities," *Family Court Review* 45, no. 3 (2007): 399–413, https://doi.org/10.1111/j.1744-1617.2007.00155.x.

8. Golightley, "Troubling the 'Troubled Teen' Industry."

9. Jennifer Greif Green et al., "School Mental Health Resources and Adolescent Mental Health Service Use," *Journal of the American Academy of Child and Adolescent Psychiatry* 52, no. 5 (2013): 501–10, https://doi.org/10.1016/j .jaac.2013.03.002.

10. *Mental Health: A Report of the Surgeon General* (1999).

CHAPTER 10

1. Kirby Deater-Deckard, Linda Ivy, and Jessica Smith, "Resilience in Gene-Environment Transactions," *Handbook of Resilience in Children*, n.d., 49–63, https://doi.org/10.1007/0-306-48572-9_4.

2. Laura Markham, *Peaceful Parent, Happy Kids: How to Stop Yelling and Start Connecting* (New York: Perigee Book, 2012).

3. Laura Markham, email message to author, June 6, 2021.

4. Foster Cline and Jim Fay, *Parenting with Love and Logic: Teaching Children Responsibility*, 3rd ed. (Colorado Springs: NavPress Publishing Group, 2014).

5. Foster Cline and Jim Fay, *Parenting Teens with Love & Logic: Preparing Adolescents for Responsible Adulthood*, 3rd ed. (Colorado Springs: NavPress, 2020).

6. Thomas Phelan, *1-2-3 Magic: Effective Discipline for Children 2–12* (Naperville, IL: Sourcebooks, 2016).

7. Ross W. Greene, *The Explosive Child: A New Approach for Understanding and Parenting Easily Frustrated, Chronically Inflexible Children* (New York: Harper, 2021).

8. Rachael C. Murrihy et al., "Community-Delivered Collaborative and Proactive Solutions and Parent Management Training for Oppositional Youth: A Randomized Trial," *Behavior Therapy* 54, no. 2 (2023): 400–17, https://doi.org/10.1016/j.beth.2022.10.005.

9. Melissa Mulraney et al., "Collaborative and Proactive Solutions Compared with Usual Care to Treat Irritability in Children and Adolescents: A Pilot Randomized Controlled Trial," *Clinical Psychologist* 26, no. 2 (2022): 231–39, https://doi.org/10.1080/13284207.2022.2041983.

10. Jacqueline Corcoran, *Living with Mental Disorder: Insights from Qualitative Research* (London: Routledge, Taylor & Francis Group, 2018).

Bibliography

aan het Rot, Marije, Sanjay J. Mathew, and Dennis S. Charney. "Neurobiological Mechanisms in Major Depressive Disorder." *Canadian Medical Association Journal* 180, no. 3 (2009), 305–13.

Abela, John R. Z., Karen Brozina, and Emily P. Haigh. "An Examination of the Response Styles Theory of Depression in Third- and Seventh-Grade Children: A Short-Term Longitudinal Study." *Journal of Abnormal Child Psychology* 30, no. 5 (2002): 515–27.

Abramson, Lyn Y., Martin E. Seligman, and John D. Teasdale. "Learned Helplessness in Humans: Critique and Reformulation." *Journal of Abnormal Psychology* 87, no. 1 (1978): 49–74.

Alexander, James, and Bruce V. Parsons. *Functional Family Therapy.* Monterey, CA: Brooks/Cole, 1982.

Alisic, Eva, et al. "Rates of Post-Traumatic Stress Disorder in Trauma-Exposed Children and Adolescents: Meta-Analysis." *British Journal of Psychiatry* 204, no. 5 (2014): 335–40. doi:10.1192/bjp.bp.113.131227.

Allen, Leila, et al. "The Correlation Between Social Support and Post-Traumatic Stress Disorder in Children and Adolescents: A Meta-Analysis." *Journal of Affective Disorders* 294 (2021): 543–57. https://doi.org/10.1016/j.jad.2021.07.028.

American Psychiatric Association, *Diagnostic and Statistical Manual of Mental Disorders*, 5th ed., text revision (DSM-5-TR) (Washington, DC: American Psychiatric Association, 2022).

Anderson, Allegra S., et al. "Parental Drug Use Disorders and Youth Psychopathology: Meta-Analytic Review." *Drug and Alcohol Dependence* 244 (2023): 109793. https://doi.org/10.1016/j.drugalcdep.2023.109793.

Arditti, Raphaël, and Yann Le Strat. "A Traumatic Life Experience in Childhood Increases the Risk of a Psychiatric Disorder in the Offspring." *Psychiatry Research* 290 (2020): 113101. https://doi.org/10.1016/j.psychres.2020.113101.

Argyriou, Angeliki, Kimberly A. Goldsmith, and Katherine A. Rimes. "Mediators of the Disparities in Depression Between Sexual Minority and Heterosexual Individuals: A Systematic Review." *Archives of Sexual Behavior* 50, no. 3 (2021): 925–59. https://doi.org/10.1007/s10508-020 -01862-0

"Autism and Developmental Disabilities Monitoring (ADDM) Network." Centers for Disease Control, n.d. https://www.cdc.gov/ncbddd/autism/pdf/ ADDM-Community-Report-SY2020-h.pdf.

Avenevoli, Shelly, et al. "Major Depression in the National Comorbidity Survey—Adolescent Supplement: Prevalence, Correlates, and Treatment." *Journal of the American Academy of Child & Adolescent Psychiatry* 54, no. 1 (2015): 37–44.

Ayano, Getinet, et al. "The Risk of Anxiety Disorders in Children of Parents with Severe Psychiatric Disorders: A Systematic Review and Meta-Analysis." *Journal of Affective Disorders* 282 (2021): 472–87. https:// doi.org/10.1016/j.jad.2020.12.134.

Baghdadli, Amaria, et al. "Developmental Trajectories of Adaptive Behaviors from Early Childhood to Adolescence in a Cohort of 152 Children with Autism Spectrum Disorders." *Journal of Autism and Developmental Disorders* 42 (2012): 1314–25. https://doi.org/10.1007/s10803-011-1357-z.

Baglivio, Michael T., et al. "The Role of Adverse Childhood Experiences (Aces) and Psychopathic Features on Juvenile Offending Criminal Careers to Age 18." *Youth Violence and Juvenile Justice* 18, no. 4 (2020): 337–64. https://doi.org/10.1177/1541204020927075.

Balakar, Jennifer L., et al. "Recent Advances in Developmental and Risk Factor Research on Eating Disorders." *Current Psychiatry Reports* 17, no. 6 (2015): 1–10. https://doi.org/10.1007/s11920-015-0585-x.

Beck, Natalie, and Jennifer S. Wong. "A Meta-Analysis of the Effects of Wilderness Therapy on Delinquent Behaviors Among Youth." *Criminal Justice and Behavior* 49, no. 5 (2022): 700–729. https://doi.org/10.21428/ cb6ab371.e81872f8.

Bégin, Vincent, et al. "Perinatal and Early-Life Factors Associated with Stable and Unstable Trajectories of Psychopathic Traits Across Childhood." *Psychological Medicine* 53, no. 2 (2023): 379–87. https://doi.org/10.1017/ s0033291721001586.

Behar, Lenore, et al. "Protecting Youth Placed in Unlicensed, Unregulated Residential 'Treatment' Facilities." *Family Court Review* 45, no. 3 (2007): 399–413. https://doi.org/10.1111/j.1744-1617.2007.00155.x.

Bekhet, Abir K., Norah L. Johnson, and Jaclene A. Zauszniewski. "Resilience in Family Members of Persons with Autism Spectrum Disorder: A Review of the Literature." *Issues in Mental Health Nursing* 33, no. 10 (2012): 650–56. https://doi.org/10.3109/01612840.2012.671441.

Berg, R. C., et al. *Interventions for Children and Youth with Behavioural Problems or Criminal Behaviour: An Overview of Reviews*. Norwegian Institute of Public Health, 2020.

Bergey, Meredith, et al. "Mapping Mental Health Inequalities: The Intersecting Effects of Gender, Race, Class, and Ethnicity on ADHD Diagnosis." *Sociology of Health & Illness* 44, no. 3 (2022): 604–23. doi:10.1111/1467-9566.13443.

Bertelsen, Thomas B., Joeseph A. Himle, and Ashlid T. Haland. "Bidirectional Relationship Between Family Accommodation and Youth Anxiety During Cognitive-Behavioral Treatment." *Child Psychiatry and Human Development* 54, no. 3 (2023): 905–12. doi:10.1007/s10578-021-01304-5.

Bettmann, Joanna E., et al. "A Meta-Analysis of Wilderness Therapy Outcomes for Private Pay Clients." *Journal of Child and Family Studies* 25, no. 9 (2016): 2659–73. https://doi.org/10.1007/s10826-016-0439-0.

Bhatara, Vinod S., Bettina Bernstein, and Sheeba Fazili. "Complementary and Integrative Treatments of Aggressiveness/Emotion Dysregulation: Associated with Disruptive Disorders and Disruptive Mood Dysregulation Disorder." *Child and Adolescent Psychiatric Clinics of North America* 32, no. 2 (2023): 297–315. https://doi.org/10.1016/j.chc.2022.08.010.

Bitsko, Rebecca H., et al. "Mental Health Surveillance Among Children—United States, 2013–2019." *Morbidity and Mortality Weekly Report* 71, no. 2 (2022): 1–48.

Bouchard, Maryse F., et al. "Attention-Deficit / Hyperactivity Disorder and Urinary Metabolites of Organophosphate Pesticides." *Pediatrics* 125, no. 6 (2010): 1270–77. https://doi.org/10.1542/peds.2009-3058.

Bouzy, Juliette, et al. "Transidentities and Autism Spectrum Disorder: A Systematic Review." *Psychiatry Research* 323 (2023): 115176. https://doi.org/10.1016/j.psychres.2023.115176.

Breaux, Rosanna, et al. "Systematic Review and Meta-Analysis: Pharmacological and Nonpharmacological Interventions for Persistent Nonepisodic Irritability." *Journal of the American Academy of Child and Adolescent Psychiatry* 62, no. 3 (2023): 318–34. https://doi.org/10.1016/j.jaac.2022.05.012.

Brown, Thomas E., and William J. McMullen. "Attention Deficit Disorders and Sleep/Arousal Disturbance." *Annals of the New York Academy of Sciences Journal* 931 (2001): 271–86. https://doi.org/10.1111/j.1749-6632.2001.tb05784.x.

Bryant-Waugh, Rachel. "Avoidant/Restrictive Food Intake Disorder." *Child and Adolescent Psychiatric Clinics of North America* 28, no. 4 (2019): 557–65. https://doi.org/10.1016/j.chc.2019.05.004.

Cairns, Kathryn E., et al. "Risk and Protective Factors for Depression That Adolescents Can Modify: A Systematic Review and Meta-Analysis of Longitudinal Studies." *Journal of Affective Disorders* 169 (2014): 61–75.

Carbonneau, Rene, et al. "Early Risk Factors Associated with Preschool Developmental Patterns of Single and Co-Occurrent Disruptive Behaviors in a Population Sample." *Developmental Psychology* 58, no. 3 (2022): 438–52. https://doi.org/10.1037/dev0001295.

Castellví, Pere, et al. "Assessing the Relationship Between School Failure and Suicidal Behavior in Adolescents and Young Adults: A Systematic Review and Meta-Analysis of Longitudinal Studies." *School Mental Health* 12, no. 3 (2020): 429–41. https://doi.org/10.1007/s12310-020-09363-0.

Centers for Disease Control and Prevention. "Disparities in Suicide." Suicide Prevention. Last modified May 2023. https://www.cdc.gov/suicide/facts/disparities-in-suicide.html.

Centers for Disease Control and Prevention. "Number and Percentage of Students, by Sexual Identity." Youth Risk Behaviors Surveys. Last reviewed April 2023. https://www.cdc.gov/healthyyouth/data/yrbs/supplemental-mmwr/students_by_sexual_identity.htm.

Centers for Disease Control and Prevention. "Youth Risk Behavior Survey Data Summary & Trends Report." Adolescent and School Health. Last reviewed April 2023. https://www.cdc.gov/healthyyouth/data/yrbs/pdf/YRBS_Data-Summary-Trends_Report2023_508.pdf.

Chan, Eugenia, Jason M. Fogler, and Paul G. Hammerness. "Treatment of Attention-Deficit/Hyperactivity Disorder in Adolescents: A Systematic Review." *Journal of American Medical Association* 315, no. 8 (2016): 1997–2008. https://doi.org/10.1001/jama.2016.5453.

Chang, Zheng, et al. "Stimulant ADHD Medication and Risk for Substance Abuse." *Journal of Child Psychology and Psychiatry* 55 (2014): 878–85. https://doi-org.proxy.library.upenn.edu/10.1111/jcpp.12164.

Chavez, Laura, et al. "Trends in Office-Based Anxiety Treatment Among US Children, Youth, and Young Adults: 2006–2018." *Pediatrics* 152, no. 1 (2023): e2022059416. 10.1542/peds.2022–059416.

Chen, L. C., et al. "Association of Parental Depression with Offspring Attention Deficit Hyperactivity Disorder and Autism Spectrum Disorder: A Nationwide Birth Cohort Study." *Journal of Affective Disorders* 277 (2020): 109–14. https://doi.org/10.1016/j.jad.2020.07.059.

"Child Maltreatment 2019: Summary of Key Findings." Child Welfare Information Gateway, n.d. https://www.childwelfare.gov/pubs/factsheets/canstats/.

Child to Parent Violence (CPV)—proceduresonline.com. Accessed June 24, 2023. https://proceduresonline.com/nesubregion/files/southtyne_cpv.pdf.

Chithiramohan, Tamara, and Guy D. Eslick. "Association Between Maternal Postnatal Depression and Offspring Anxiety and Depression in Adolescence and Young Adulthood: A Meta-Analysis." *Journal of Developmental &*

Behavioral Pediatrics 44, no. 3 (2023): e231–e238. https://doi.org/10.1097/DBP.0000000000001164.

Choi, Won-Jun, et al. "Blood Lead, Parental Marital Status and the Risk of Attention-Deficit/Hyperactivity Disorder in Elementary School Children: A Longitudinal Study." *Psychiatry Research* 236 (2016): 42–46. https://doi.org/10.1016/j.psychres.2016.01.002.

Cipriana, Annarosa, Stefania Cella, and Paolo Cotrufo. "Nonsuicidal Self-Injury A Systematic Review." *Frontiers in Psychology* (November 2017). doi: 10.3389/fpsyg.2017.01946.

Cipriani, Andrea, et al. "Comparative Efficacy and Tolerability of Antidepressants for Major Depressive Disorder in Children and Adolescents: A Network Meta-Analysis." *The Lancet* (British Edition) 388 (100477), June 2016: 881–90. https://doi.org/10.1016/S0140-6736(16)30385-3.

Clarke, Greg N., P. M. Lewinsohn, and H. Hops. "Adolescent Coping with Depression Course. Kaiser Permanente." *Kaiser Permanente Center for Health Research* (1990). http://www.kpchr.org/acwd/acwd.html.

Cline, Foster, and Jim Fay. *Parenting with Love and Logic: Teaching Children Responsibility.* Carol Stream, IL: NavPress Publishing Group, 2020.

Cline, Foster, and Jim Fay. *Parenting Teens with Love & Logic: Preparing Adolescents for Responsible Adulthood.* 3rd ed. Colorado Springs: NavPress, 2020.

Cohen, Judith A., Esther Deblinger, and Anthony P. Mannarino. *Treating Trauma and Traumatic Grief in Children and Adolescents.* 2nd ed. New York: Guilford Press, 2017.

Coley, Rebekah Levine, et al. "A Quasi-Experimental Evaluation of Marijuana Policies and Youth Marijuana Use." *American Journal of Drug and Alcohol Abuse* 45, no. 3 (2019): 292–303. https://doi.org/10.1080/00952990.2018.1559847.

Connor, Daniel F., Jennifer Steeber, and Keith McBurnett. "A Review of Attention-Deficit/Hyperactivity Disorder Complicated by Symptoms of Oppositional Defiant Disorder or Conduct Disorder." *Journal of Developmental and Behavioral Pediatrics* 31 (2010): 427–40. https://doi.org/10.1097/DBP.0b013e3181e121bd.

Corcoran, Jacqueline. *Living with Mental Disorder: Insights from Qualitative Research.* London: Routledge, Taylor & Francis Group, 2018.

Corcoran, Jacqueline, and Joseph Walsh. *Clinical Assessment and Diagnosis in Social Work Practice.* 4th ed. New York: Oxford University Press, 2022.

Corcoran, Jacqueline, et al. "Parents of Children with Attention Deficit/Hyperactivity Disorder: A Meta-Synthesis, Part I." *Child and Adolescent Social Work Journal* 34 (2017): 281–335. DOI: 10.1007/s10560-016-0465-1.

Corcoran, Jacqueline, et al. "Parents of Children with Attention Deficit/ Hyperactivity Disorder: A Meta-Synthesis, Part II." *Child and Adolescent Social Work Journal* 34 (2017): 337–48. DOI: 10.1007/s10560-017-0497-1.

Cordova, Michaela M., et al. "Attention-Deficit/Hyperactivity Disorder: Restricted Phenotypes Prevalence, Comorbidity, and Polygenic Risk Sensitivity in the ABCD Baseline Cohort." *Journal of the American Academy of Child & Adolescent Psychiatry* 61, no. 10 (2022): 1273–84. https://doi.org/10.1016/j.jaac.2022.03.030.

Correll, Christoph U., et al. "Efficacy and Acceptability of Pharmacological, Psychosocial, and Brain Stimulation Interventions in Children and Adolescents with Mental Disorders: An Umbrella Review." *World Psychiatry* 20, no. 2 (2021): 244–75. https://doi.org/10.1002/wps.20881.

Cortese, Samuele, et al. "Comparative Efficacy and Tolerability of Medications for Attention-Deficit Hyperactivity Disorder in Children, Adolescents, and Adults: A Systematic Review and Network Meta-Analysis." *The Lancet* 5, no. 9 (2018): 727–38. https://doi.org/10.1016/S2215-0366(18)30269-4.

Couturier, Jennifer, et al. "Psychotropic Medication for Children and Adolescents with Eating Disorders." *Child and Adolescent Psychiatric Clinics of North America* 28, no. 4 (2019): 583–92. https://doi.org/10.1016 /j.chc.2019.05.005.

Craig, Francesco, et al. "A Systematic Review of Coping Strategies in Parents of Children with Attention Deficit Hyperactivity Disorder (ADHD). *Research in Developmental Disabilities* 98 (2020): 103571. https://doi.org/10.1016/j .ridd.2020.103571.

Craig, S. G., N. Goulter, and M. M. Moretti. "A Systematic Review of Primary and Secondary Callous-Unemotional Traits and Psychopathy Variants in Youth." *Clinical Child and Family Psychology Review* 24, no. 1 (2020): 65–91. https://doi.org/10.1007/s10567-020-00329-x.

Craig, Stephanie G., et al. "The Mediational Effect of Affect Dysregulation on the Association Between Attachment to Parents and Oppositional Defiant Disorder Symptoms in Adolescents." *Child Psychiatry and Human Development* 52, no. 5 (2020): 818–28. https://doi.org/10.1007/s10578-020 -01059-5.

Cramer, J., and P. Wanner. "Wilderness Therapy Programs: A Systematic Review of Research, June 2022." https://www.wsipp.wa.gov/ReportFile /1748/Wsipp_Wilderness-Therapy-Programs-A-Systematic-Review-of -Research_Report.pdf.

Dachew, Berihun Assefa, et al. "Association of Maternal Depressive Symptoms During the Perinatal Period with Oppositional Defiant Disorder in Children and Adolescents." *JAMA Network Open* 4, no. 9 (2021). https://doi.org/10 .1001/jamanetworkopen.2021.25854.

Dalle Grave, Riccardo, Massimiliano Sartirana, and Simona Calugi. "Enhanced Cognitive Behavioral Therapy for Adolescents with Anorexia Nervosa: Outcomes and Predictors of Change in a Real-World Setting." *International Journal of Eating Disorders* 52, no. 9 (2019): 1042–46. https://doi.org/10.1002/eat.23122.

Dane, Alexandra, and Komal Bhatia. "The Social Media Diet: A Scoping Review to Investigate the Association Between Social Media, Body Image and Eating Disorders Amongst Young People." *PLOS Global Public Health* 3, no. 3 (2023). https://doi.org/10.1371/journal.pgph.0001091.

Daniels, Amy M., and David S. Mandell. "Explaining Differences in Age at Autism Spectrum Disorder Diagnosis: A Critical Review." *Autism* 18, no. 5 (2013): 583–97. https://doi.org/10.1177/1362361313480277.

Danielson, Melissa L., et al. "Prevalence of Parent-Reported ADHD Diagnosis and Associated Treatment Among U.S. Children and Adolescents, 2016." *Journal of Clinical Child and Adolescent Psychology* 47, no. 2 (2018): 199–212. http://doi.org/10.1080/15374416.2017.1417860

Datta, Nandini, et al. "Evidence Based Update on Psychosocial Treatments for Eating Disorders in Children and Adolescents." *Official Journal for the Society of Clinical Child and Adolescent Psychology, American Psychological Association* 52, no. 2 (2023): 159–70. https://doi.org/10.1080/15374416.2022.2109650.

Davey, Emily, et al. "'It Opened My Eyes': Parents' Experiences of Their Child Receiving an Anxiety Disorder Diagnosis." *Clinical Child Psychology and Psychiatry* 27, no. 3 (2022): 658–69. doi:10.1177/13591045221088708.

Deater-Deckard, Kirby, Linda Ivy, and Jessica Smith. "Resilience in Gene-Environment Transactions." *Handbook of Resilience in Children*, n.d., 49–63. https://doi.org/10.1007/0-306-48572-9_4.

Deconinck, Nicolas, Marie Soncarrieu, and Bernard Dan. "Toward Better Recognition of Early Predictors for Autism Spectrum Disorders." *Pediatric Neurology* 49, no. 4 (2013): 225–31. https://doi.org/10.1016/j.pediatrneurol.2013.05.012.

Dekkers, Tycho J., et al. "Decision-Making Deficits in Adolescent Boys with and without Attention-Deficit/Hyperactivity Disorder (ADHD): An Experimental Assessment of Associated Mechanisms." *Journal of Abnormal Child Psychology* 48, no. 4 (2020): 495–510. https://doi.org/10.1007/s10802-019-00613-7.

Dekkers, Tycho J., et al. "The Importance of Parental Knowledge in the Association Between ADHD Symptomatology and Related Domains of Impairment." *European Journal of Child Adolescent Psychiatry* 30, no. 4 (2021): 657–69. https://doi.org/10.1007/s00787-020-01579-4.

Dekkers, Tycho J., et al. "Meta-Analysis: Which Components of Parent Training Work for Children with Attention-Deficit/Hyperactivity Disorder?" *Journal of the American Academy of Child & Adolescent Psychiatry* 61, no. 4 (2022): 478–94. https://doi.org/10.1016/j.jaac.2021.06.015

DeVita-Raeburn, Elizabeth, and Spectrum. "Is the Most Common Therapy for Autism Cruel?" *The Atlantic*, August 12, 2016. https://www.theatlantic.com /health/archive/2016/08/aba-autism-controversy/495272/.

Dimidjian, Sona, et al. "The Origins and Current Status of Behavioral Activation Treatments for Depression." *Annual Review of Clinical Psychology* 7 (January 2011): 1–38. https://doi.org/10.1146/annurev-clinpsy-032210 -104535.

Donohue, Brad, et al. "Family Behavior Therapy for Substance Abuse and Other Associated Problems." *Behavior Modification* 33, no. 5 (2009): 495–519. https://doi.org/10.1177/0145445509340019.

Dunn, Erin C., et al. "Research Review: Gene-Environment Interaction Research in Youth Depression—A Systematic Review with Recommendations for Future Research." *Journal of Child Psychology and Psychiatry* 52, no. 12 (2011): 1223–38.

Earle, Jason F. "An Introduction to the Psychopharmacology of Children and Adolescents with Autism Spectrum Disorder." *Journal of Child and Adolescent Psychiatric Nursing* 29, no. 2 (2016): 62–71. https://doi.org/10 .1111/jcap.12144.

Eckshtain, Dikla, et al. "Meta-Analysis: 13-Year Follow-up of Psychotherapy Effects on Youth Depression." *Journal of the American Academy of Child and Adolescent Psychiatry* 59 (2020): 45–63.

Egger, Helen Link, and Adrian Angold. "Common Emotional and Behavioral Disorders in Preschool Children: Presentation, Nosology, and Epidemiology." *Journal of Child Psychology and Psychiatry* 47, no. 3–4 (2006): 313–37. https://doi.org/10.1111/j.1469-7610.2006.01618.x.

Elfine, John. "Percent of Teenagers in the U.S. Taking Antidepressants from 2015 to 2019, by Gender." Statista, July 2020. https://www.statista.com/statistics /1133612/antidepressant-use-teenagers-by-gender-us/#statisticContainer.

Emerson, Natacha D., Holly E. Morrell, and Cameron Neece. "Predictors of Age of Diagnosis for Children with Autism Spectrum Disorder: The Role of a Consistent Source of Medical Care, Race, and Condition Severity." *Journal of Autism and Developmental Disorders* 46, no. 1 (2016): 127–38. https://doi.org/10.1007/s10803-015-2555-x.

Espinosa, Fabiola, Nuria Martin-Romero, and Alvaro Sanchez-Lopez. "Repetitive Negative Thinking Processes Account for Gender Differences in Depression and Anxiety During Adolescence." *International Journal of Cognitive Therapy* 15, no. 2 (2022), 115–33. https://doi.org/10.1007/s41811 -022-00133-1.

Evans, Steven W., Julie S. Owens, and Nora Bunford. "Evidence-Based Psychosocial Treatments for Children and Adolescents with Attention-Deficit/

Hyperactivity Disorder." *Journal of Clinical Child and Adolescent Psychology* 43, no. 4 (2014): 527–51. https://doi.org/10.1080/15374416.2013.850700.

"F&D Basic Materials." Friendships & Dating Program, n.d. https://www.fdprogram.org/store/p1/F%26D_Basic_Materials.html.

Fabiano, Gregory A., and Kellina Pyle. "Best Practices in School Mental Health for Attention-Deficit/Hyperactivity Disorder: A Framework for Intervention." *School Mental Health* 11, no. 1 (2019): 72–91. https://doi.org /10.1007/s12310-018-9267-2.

Fadus, Matthew C., et al. "Unconscious Bias and the Diagnosis of Disruptive Behavior Disorders and ADHD in African American and Hispanic Youth." *Academic Psychiatry* 44, no. 1 (2020): 95–102. https://doi.org/10.1007/ s40596-019-01127-6.

Fagan, Abigail A. "Child Maltreatment and Aggressive Behaviors in Early Adolescence: Evidence of Moderation by Parent/Child Relationship Quality." *Child Maltreatment* 25, no. 2 (2019): 182–91. https://doi.org/10 .1177/1077559519874401.

Fazel, Seena, Helen Doll, and Niklas Langstrom. "Mental Disorders Among Adolescents in Juvenile Detention and Correctional Facilities: A Systematic Review and Metaregression Analysis of 25 Surveys." *Journal of the American Academy of Child and Adolescent Psychiatry* 47, no. 9 (2008): 1010–19.

Filipponi, Caterina, et al. "The Follow-Up of Eating Disorders from Adolescence to Early Adulthood: A Systematic Review." *International Journal of Environmental Research and Public Health* 19, no. 23 (2022): 16237. https: //doi.org/10.3390/ijerph192316237.

Finer, Lawrence B., and Mira R. Zolna. "Declines in Unintended Pregnancy in the United States, 2008–2011." *New England Journal of Medicine* 374, no. 9 (2016): 843–52. https://doi.org/10.1056/NEJMsa1506575.

Flaherty, Colleen. "Mental Health Crisis for Grad Students." *Inside Higher Ed* (2018).

Fox, Nathan A., et al. "Annual Research Review: Developmental Pathways Linking Early Behavioral Inhibition to Later Anxiety." *Journal of Child Psychology and Psychiatry* 64, no. 4 (2023): 537–61. doi:10.1111/jcpp.13702.

Friedman, J., et al. "Trends in Drug Overdose Deaths Among US Adolescents, January 2010 to June 2021." *JAMA* 327, no. 14 (2022): 1398–1400. doi:10.1001/jama.2022.2847.

Friedman, Keren, et al. "A Narrative Review of Outcome Studies for Residential and Partial Hospital-Based Treatment of Eating Disorders." *Journal of the Eating Disorders Association* 24, no. 4 (2016): 263–76. https: //doi.org/10.1002/erv.2449.

Furzer, Jill, Elizabeth Dhuey, and Audrey Laporte. "ADHD Misdiagnosis: Causes and Mitigators." *Health Economics* 31, no 9 (2022): 1926–53. https://doi.org/10.1002/hec.4555.

Garner, David M., et al. "Psychotropic Medications in Adult and Adolescent Eating Disorders: Clinical Practice versus Evidence-Based Recommendations." *Eating and Weight Disorders—Studies on Anorexia, Bulimia and Obesity* 21, no. 3 (2016): 395–402. https://doi.org/10.1007/s40519-016-0253-0.

Gates, Jacquelyn A., Erin Kang, and Matthew D. Lerner. "Efficacy of Group Social Skills Interventions for Youth with Autism Spectrum Disorder: A Systematic Review and Meta-Analysis." *Clinical Psychology Review* 52 (2017): 164–81. https://doi.org/10.1016/j.cpr.2017.01.006.

Ghandour, Reem M., et al. "Prevalence and Treatment of Depression, Anxiety, and Conduct Problems in US Children." *Journal of Pediatrics* (2020). doi: 10.1016/j.jpeds.2018.09.021.

Gilbert, Kirsten, et al. "Childhood Behavioral Inhibition and Overcontrol: Relationships with Cognitive Functioning, Error Monitoring, Anxiety and Obsessive-Compulsive Symptoms." *Research on Child and Adolescent Psychopathology* 50, no. 12 (2022): 1629–42. doi:10.1007/s10802-022-00953-x.

Gillies, Donna, et al. "Prevalence and Characteristics of Self-Harm in Adolescents: Meta-Analyses of Community-Based Studies 1990–2015." *Journal of the American Academy of Child & Adolescent Psychiatry* (October 2018). doi: 10.1016/j.jaac.2018.06.018.

Gizer, Ian R., Courtney Ficks, and Irwin D. Waldman. "Candidate Gene Studies of ADHD: A Meta-Analytic Review." *Human Genetics* 126 (2009): 51–90. https://doi.org/10.1007/s00439-009-0694-x.

Glasofer, Amy, Catherine Dingley, and Andrew T. Reyes. "Medication Decision Making Among African American Caregivers of Children with ADHD: A Review of Literature." *Journal of Attention Disorders* 25, no. 12 (2021): 1687–98. https://doi.org/10.1177/1087054720930783.

Golden, Neville H., et al. "Position Paper of the Society for Adolescent Health and Medicine: Medical Management of Restrictive Eating Disorders in Adolescents and Young Adults." *Journal of Adolescent Health* 56, no. 1 (2015): 121–25.

Golightley, Sarah. "Troubling the 'Troubled Teen' Industry: Adult Reflections on Youth Experiences of Therapeutic Boarding Schools." *Global Studies of Childhood* 10, no. 1 (2020): 53–63. https://doi.org/10.1177/2043610619900514.

Goodman, Sherryl H., et al. "Parenting As a Mediator of Associations Between Depression in Mothers and Children's Functioning: A Systematic Review and Meta-Analysis." *Clinical Child and Family Psychology Review* (July

2020). https://doi-org.proxy.library.upenn.edu/10.1007/s10567-020-00322 -4.

Goodman, Sherryl H., and Judy Garber. "Evidence-Based Interventions for Depression Mothers and Their Young Children." *Child Development Journal* (March 2017). doi: 10.1111/cdev.12732

Graves, Tiffany A., et al. "A Meta-Analysis of the Relation Between Therapeutic Alliance and Treatment Outcome in Eating Disorders." *International Journal of Eating Disorders* 50, no. 4 (2017): 323–40. https://doi.org/10 .1002/eat.22672.

Gray, Carol, and Barry M. Prizant. *The New Social Story Book*. Arlington, TX: Future Horizons, 2015.

Green, Jennifer Greif, et al. "School Mental Health Resources and Adolescent Mental Health Service Use." *Journal of the American Academy of Child and Adolescent Psychiatry* 52, no. 5 (2013): 501–10. https://doi.org/10.1016/j .jaac.2013.03.002.

Greene, Ross. *The Explosive Child: A New Approach for Understanding and Parenting Easily Frustrated, Chronically Inflexible Children*. New York: Harper, 2021.

Greenhill, Laurence L., et al. "Trajectories of Growth Associated with Long-Term Stimulant Medication in the Multimodal Treatment Study of Attention-Deficit/Hyperactivity Disorder." *Journal of the American Academy of Child & Adolescent Psychiatry* 59, no. 8 (2020): 978–89. https: //doi.org/10.1016/j.jaac.2019.06.019.

Grimmond, Jessica, et al. "A Qualitative Systematic Review of Experiences and Perceptions of Youth Suicide." *PLOS One* (2019). doi: 10.1371/journal. pone.0217569.

Gryczkowski, Michelle R., and Stephen P. H. Whiteside. "Pediatric Obsessive-Compulsive Disorder," in *Obsessive-Compulsive Disorder and Its Spectrum: A Life-Span Approach,* E. A. Storch and D. McKay, eds., 37–57. Washington, DC: American Psychological Association, 2014.

Guideline Development Panel for the Treatment of Depressive Disorders. "Summary of the Clinical Practice Guideline for the Treatment of Depression Across Three Age Cohorts." American Psychologist 77, no. 6 (2022): 770– 80. https://doi.org/10.1037/amp0000904.

Guina, Jeffrey, et al. "Should Posttraumatic Stress Be a Disorder or a Specifier? Towards Improved Nosology within the DSM Categorical Classification System." *Current Psychiatry Reports* 19, no. 66 (2017). https://doi.org/10 .1007/s11920-017-0821-7.

Haan, Elis, et al. "Prenatal Smoking, Alcohol and Caffeine Exposure and Maternal-Reported Attention Deficit Hyperactivity Disorder Symptoms in Childhood: Triangulation of Evidence Using Negative Control and

Polygenic Risk Score Analyses." *Addiction* 117, no. 5 (2022): 1458–71. https://doi.org/10.1111/add.15746.

Haasz, Maya, et al. "Firearms Availability Among High-School Age Youth with Recent Depression or Suicidality." *Pediatrics* 151, no. 6 (2023): 1.

Hall, William. "Psychosocial Risk and Protective Factors for Depression Among Lesbian, Gay, Bisexual, and Queer Youth: A Systematic Review." *Journal of Homosexuality* 65, no. 3 (2018): 263–316. doi: 10.1080/00918369.2017.1317467.

Hambly, Jessica L., et al. "Pharmacotherapy of Conduct Disorder: Challenges, Options and Future Directions." *Journal of Psychopharmacology* 30, no. 10 (2016): 967–75. https://doi.org/10.1177/0269881116658985.

Hancock, Grace I., Mark A. Stokes, and Gary B. Mesibov. "Socio-Sexual Functioning in Autism Spectrum Disorder: A Systematic Review and Meta-Analyses of Existing Literature." *Autism Research* 10, no. 11 (2017): 1823–33. https://doi.org/10.1002/aur.1831.

Hangül, Zehra, and Ali Evren Tufan. "Use of Complementary and Alternative Therapies in Autism Spectrum Disorder." *Psikiyatride Güncel Yaklaşımlar* 14, no. 2 (2022): 165–73. https://doi.org/10.18863/pgy.935207.

Harrington, Anne. *Mind Fixers: Psychiatry's Troubled Search for the Biology of Mental Illness*. New York: W.W. Norton & Company, 2020.

Harris, Gardiner. "Drug Maker Told Studies Would Aid It, Papers Say." *New York Times*, March 19, 2009.

Harris, Gardiner. "Research Center Tied to Drug Company." *New York Times*, November 24, 2008.

Harris, Gardiner, and Benedict Carey. "Researchers Fail to Reveal Full Drug Pay." *New York Times*, June 8, 2008.

Hart, Heledd, et al. "Meta-Analysis of Functional Magnetic Resonance Imaging Studies of Inhibition and Attention in Attention-Deficit/ Hyperactivity Disorder: Exploring Task-Specific, Stimulant Medication, and Age Effects." *Journal of American Medical Association Psychiatry* 70, no. 2 (2013): 185–98. https://doi.org/10.1001/jamapsychiatry.2013.277.

Hathorn, Claire, et al. "Impact of Adherence to Best Practice Guidelines on the Diagnostic and Assessment Services for Autism Spectrum Disorder." *Journal of Autism and Developmental Disorders* 44, no. 8 (2014): 1859–66. https://doi.org/10.1007/s10803-014-2057-2.

Hawton, Keith, et al. "Risk Factors for Suicide in Individuals with Depression: A Systematic Review." *Journal of Affective Disorders* (2013). doi: 10.1016/j.jad.2013.01.004.

Hemmingsen, C. H., et al. "Maternal Use of Hormonal Contraception and Risk of Childhood ADHD: A Nationwide Population-Based Cohort Study. *European Journal of Epidemiology* 35, no. 9 (2020): 795–805. https://doi.org/10.1007/s10654-020-00673-w.

Henderson, Ziporah B., et al. "Emotional Development in Eating Disorders: A Qualitative Metasynthesis." *Clinical Psychology & Psychotherapy* 26, no. 4 (2019): 440–57. https://doi.org/10.1002/cpp.2365.

Henneberger, Angela K., Dawnsha R. Mushonga, and Alison M. Preston. "Peer Influence and Adolescent Substance Use: A Systematic Review of Dynamic Social Network Research." *Adolescent Research Review* 6, no. 1 (2021): 57–73. https://doi.org/10.1007/s40894-019-00130-0.

Hetrick, Sarah E., et al. "New Generation Antidepressants for Depression in Children and Adolescents: A Network Meta-Analysis." *Cochrane Library* (May 2021). https://doi.org/10.1002/14651858.CD013674.pub2.

Hicks, Brian M., et al. "Environmental Adversity and Increasing Genetic Risk for Externalizing Disorders." *Archives of General Psychiatry* 66, no. 6 (2009): 640–48. https://doi.org/10.1001/archgenpsychiatry.2008.554.

Hidalgo, Nina Jamilette, et al. "Sociodemographic Differences in Parental Satisfaction with an Autism Spectrum Disorder Diagnosis." *Journal of Intellectual and Developmental Disability* 40, no. 2 (2015): 147–55. https://doi.org/10.3109/13668250.2014.994171.

Higa-McMillan, Charmaine K., et al. "Evidence Base Update: 50 Years of Research on Treatment for Child and Adolescent Anxiety." *Journal of Clinical Child and Adolescent Psychology* 45, no. 2 (2016): 91–113. doi:10.1080/15374416.2015.1046177.

Hiller, Rachel M., et al. "A Longitudinal Investigation of the Role of Parental Responses in Predicting Children's Post-Traumatic Distress." *Journal of Child Psychology and Psychiatry* 59, no. 7 (2018): 781–89. https://doi.org/10.1111/jcpp.12846.

Hillman, Kylie, et al. *Interventions for Anxiety in Mainstream School-Aged Children with Autism Spectrum Disorder: A Systematic Review.* Hoboken, NJ: John Wiley & Sons, 2020.

Hinshaw, Stephen. "Attention Deficit Hyperactivity Disorder (ADHD): Controversy, Developmental Mechanisms, and Multiple Levels of Analysis." *Annual Review of Clinical Psychology* 14 (2018): 291–316. https://doi.org/10.1146/annurev-clinpsy-050817-084917.

Hirota, Tomoya, et al. "Antiepileptic Medications in Autism Spectrum Disorder: A Systematic Review and Meta-Analysis." *Journal of Autism and Developmental Disorders* 44, no. 4 (2014): 948–57. https://doi.org/10.1007/s10803-013-1952-2.

Hoare, Erin, et al. "The Associations Between Sedentary Behavior and Mental Health Among Adolescents: A Systematic Review." *International Journal of Behavioral Nutrition and Physical Activity* 13, no. 1 (2016).

Hogue, Aaron, et al. "Core Elements of CBT for Adolescent Conduct and Substance Use Problems: Comorbidity, Clinical Techniques, and Case

Examples." *Cognitive and Behavioral Practice* 27, no. 4 (2020): 426–41. https://doi.org/10.1016/j.cbpra.2019.12.002.

Hogue, Aaron, et al. "Evidence Base on Outpatient Behavioral Treatments for Adolescent Substance Use: Updates and Recommendations 2007–2013." *Journal of Clinical Child & Adolescent Psychology* 43, no. 5 (2018): 695–720. https://doi.org/10.1080/15374416.2014.915550.

Hong, C., et al. "Global Trends and Regional Differences in the Burden of Anxiety Disorders and Major Depressive Disorder Attributed to Bullying Victimisation in 204 Countries and Territories, 1999–2019: An Analysis of the Global Burden of Disease Study." *Epidemiology and Psychiatric Sciences* 31 (2022): e85. doi:10.1017/S2045796022000683.

Hopper, Christian J., Thomas J. Crowley, and John K. Hewitt. "Review of Twin and Adoption Studies of Adolescent Substance Use." *Journal of the American Academy of Child & Adolescent Psychiatry* 42, no. 6 (2003): 710–19. https://doi.org/10.1097/01.chi.0000046848.56865.54.

Hughes, Michelle M., et al. "The Prevalence and Characteristics of Children with Profound Autism, 15 Sites, United States, 2000–2016." *Public Health Reports*, 2023, 003335492311635. https://doi.org/10.1177/00333549231163551.

Humble, Jaxon J., et al. "Child-Centered Play Therapy for Youths Who Have Experienced Trauma: A Systematic Literature Review." *Journal of Child & Adolescent Trauma* 12, no. 3 (2018): 365–75. https://doi.org/10.1007/s40653-018-0235-7.

Hyde, Janet, and Amy H. Mezulis. "Gender Differences in Depression: Biological, Affective, Cognitive, and Sociocultural Factors." *Harvard Review of Psychiatry* 28, no. 1 (2020): 4–13. https://doi.org/10.1097/HRP.0000000000000230.

"Identity-First Language." Autistic Self Advocacy Network, n.d. https://autisticadvocacy.org/about-asan/identity-first-language/.

In a Different Key: The Story of Autism. PBS, 2013. https://www.pbs.org/show/different-key/.

International Society for the Study of Self-Injury. "What Is Self-Injury?" About Self-Injury. Last reviewed 2018. https://www.itriples.org/what-is-nssi

Javdani, Shabnam, McKenzie N. Berezin, and Keisha April. "A Treatment-to-Prison-Pipeline? Scoping Review and Multimethod Examination of Legal Consequences of Residential Treatment Among Adolescents." *Journal of Clinical Child & Adolescent Psychology* 52, no. 3 (2023): 376–95. https://doi.org/10.1080/15374416.2023.2178003.

Jewell, C., A. Wittkowski, and D. Pratt. "The Impact of Parent-Only Interventions on Child Anxiety: A Systematic Review and Meta-Analysis." *Journal of Affective Disorders* 309 (2022): 324–49. doi:10.1016/j.jad.2022.04.082.

Ji, Xiao, et al. "Increased Burden of Deleterious Variants in Essential Genes in Autism Spectrum Disorder." *Proceedings of the National Academy of Sciences* 113, no. 52 (2016): 15054–59. https://doi.org/10.1073/pnas .1613195113.

John, Ann, et al. "Self-Harm, Suicidal Behaviors, and Cyberbullying in Children and Young People: Systematic Review." *Journal of Medical Internet Research* (2018). doi: 10.2196/jmir.9044.

Johnson, Katherine A., Jan R. Wiersema, and Jonna Kuntsi. "What Would Karl Popper Say? Are Current Psychological Theories of ADHD Falsifiable?" *Behavioral and Brain Functions* 5, no. 15 (2009): 1–11. https: //doi.org/10.1186/1744-9081-5-15.

Jordan, Ashly E., et al. "Past-Year Prevalence of Prescription Opioid Misuse Among Those 11 to 30 Years of Age in the United States: A Systematic Review and Meta-Analysis." *Journal of Substance Abuse Treatment* 77 (2017): 31–37. https://doi.org/10.1016/j.jsat.2017.03.007.

Karniski, Walt. *ADHD Medication: Does It Work and Is It Safe?* Lanham, MD: Rowman & Littlefield, 2022.

Kearns, Jaclyn C., et al. "Sleep Problems and Suicide Risk in Youth: A Systematic Review, Developmental Framework, and Implications for Hospital Treatment. *General Hospital Psychiatry* 63 (2020): 141–51. https: //doi.org/10.1016/j.genhosppsych.2018.09.011

Kessel, Ellen M., et al. "Early Predictors of Adolescent Irritability." *Child and Adolescent Psychiatric Clinics of North America* 30, no. 3 (2021): 475–90. https://doi.org/10.1016/j.chc.2021.04.002.

Kim, Jae H., et al. "Environmental Risk Factors, Protective Factors, and Peripheral Biomarkers for ADHD: An Umbrella Review." *The Lancet* 7, no. 11 (2020): 955–70. https://doi.org/10.1016/S2215-0366(20)30312-6.

Kim, Seongju, and Dohyung Kim. "Behavioral Symptoms of Child Mental Disorders and Lifetime Substance Use in Adolescence: A Within-Family Comparison of US Siblings." *Drug and Alcohol Dependence* 219 (2021): 108490. https://doi.org/10.1016/j.drugalcdep.2020.108490.

Kirk, Stuart A., Tomi Gomory, and David Cohen. *Mad Science: Psychiatric Coercion, Diagnosis, and Drugs.* Philadelphia, PA: Routledge, 2017.

Klein, Daniel N., et al. "A Transdiagnostic Perspective on Youth Irritability." *Current Directions in Psychological Science* 30, no. 5 (2021): 437–43. https: //doi.org/10.1177/09637214211035101.

Kossowsky, Joe, et al. "The Separation Anxiety Hypothesis of Panic Disorder Revisited: A Meta-Analysis." *American Journal of Psychiatry* 170, no. 7 (2013): 768–81. doi:10.1176.appi.ajp.2012.12070893.

Kothgassner, Oswald D., et al. "Efficacy of Dialectical Behavior Therapy for Adolescent Self-Harm and Suicidal Ideation: A Systematic Review and

Meta-Analysis." *Psychological Medicine* 51, no. 7 (2021): 1057–67. https://doi.org/10.1017/S0033291721001355.

Lai, Meng-Chuan, et al. "Prevalence of Co-Occurring Mental Health Diagnoses in the Autism Population: A Systematic Review and Meta-Analysis." *The Lancet Psychiatry* 6, no. 10 (2019): 819–29. https://doi.org/10.1016/s2215-0366(19)30289-5.

Larsen, Pernille Stemann, et al. "Parental and Child Characteristics Related to Early-Onset Disordered Eating." *Harvard Review of Psychiatry* 18, no. 3 (2015): 183–202. https://doi.org/10.1097/hrp.0000000000000073.

Layton, Timothy J., et al. "Attention Deficit–Hyperactivity Disorder and Month of School Enrollment." *New England Journal of Medicine* 379, no. 22 (2018): 2122–30. https://doi.org/10.1056/NEJMoa1806828.

Le Grange, Daniel, et al. "Randomized Clinical Trial of Family-Based Treatment and Cognitive-Behavioral Therapy for Adolescent Bulimia Nervosa." *Journal of the American Academy of Child & Adolescent Psychiatry* 54, no. 11 (2015). https://doi.org/10.1016/j.jaac.2015.08.008.

Lee, Phyllis, and Jason M. Lang. "Comparing Trauma-Focused Cognitive-Behavioral Therapy to Commonly Used Treatments in Usual Care for Children with Posttraumatic Stress Disorder." *Psychological Trauma: Theory, Research, Practice, and Policy*, 2023. https://doi.org/10.1037/tra0001555.

Levin, Aaron. "Early Life Trauma Changes Biology of Brain." *Psychiatric News* 54, no. 14 (2019). https://doi.org/10.1176/appi.pn.2019.6b19.

Liang, Jing-Hong, et al. "Effectiveness Comparisons of Various Psychosocial Therapies for Children and Adolescents with Depression: A Bayesian Network Meta-Analysis." *European Child & Adolescent Psychiatry* 30, no. 5 (2021): 685–97. https://doi.org/10.1007/s00787-020-01492-w.

Liddle, Howard A., et al. "Multidimensional Family Therapy for Adolescent Drug Abuse: Results of a Randomized Clinical Trial." *American Journal of Drug and Alcohol Abuse* 27, no. 4 (2001): 651–88. https://doi.org/10.1081/ada-100107661.

Lilenfeld, Lisa R. R., et al. "Eating Disorders and Personality: A Methodological and Empirical Review." *Clinical Psychology Review* 26, no. 3 (2006): 299–320. https://doi.org/10.1016/j.cpr.2005.10.003.

Lim, Carmen C., et al. "Prevalence of Adolescent Cannabis Vaping." *JAMA Pediatrics* 176, no. 1 (2022): 42–51. https://doi.org/10.1001/jamapediatrics.2021.4102.

Lin, Xiuyun, et al. "A Systematic Review of Multiple Family Factors Associated with Oppositional Defiant Disorder." *International Journal of Environmental Research and Public Health* 19, no. 17 (2022): 10866. https://doi.org/10.3390/ijerph191710866.

Linehan, Marsha M. *Cognitive Behavioral Treatment of Borderline Personality Disorder*. New York: Guilford Press, 1993.

Liu, Mingli, Lang Wu, and Shuqiao Yao. "Dose–Response Association of Screen Time-Based Sedentary Behaviour in Children and Adolescents and Depression: A Meta-Analysis of Observational Studies." *British Journal of Sports Medicine* 50, no. 20 (2016): 1252–58.

Liu, Richard T., et al. "Prevalence and Correlates of Non-Suicidal Self-Injury Among Lesbian, Gay, Bisexual, and Transgender Individuals: A Systematic Review and Meta-Analysis." *Clinical Psychology Review* (December 2019). doi: 10.1016/j.cpr.2019.101783.

LoBraico, Emily J., et al. "Constellations of Family Risk for Long-Term Adolescent Antisocial Behavior." *Journal of Family Psychology* 34, no. 5 (2020): 587–97. https://doi.org/10.1037/fam0000640.

Lochman, John E., et al. "Cognitive-Behavioral Therapy for Externalizing Disorders in Children and Adolescents." *Child and Adolescent Psychiatric Clinics of North America* 20, no. 2 (2011): 305–18. https://doi.org/10.1016/j.chc.2011.01.005.

Lock, James. "Updates on Treatments for Adolescent Anorexia Nervosa." *Child and Adolescent Psychiatric Clinics of North America* 28, no. 4 (2019): 523–35. https://doi.org/10.1016/j.chc.2019.05.001.

Lock, James, and Daniel Le Grange. "Family-Based Treatment: Where Are We and Where Should We Be Going to Improve Recovery in Child and Adolescent Eating Disorders." *International Journal of Eating Disorders* 52, no. 4 (2018): 481–87. https://doi.org/10.1002/eat.22980.

Lock, James, and Maria C. La Via. "Practice Parameter for the Assessment and Treatment of Children and Adolescents with Eating Disorders." *Journal of the American Academy of Child & Adolescent Psychiatry* 54, no. 5 (2015): 412–25. https://doi.org/10.1016/j.jaac.2015.01.018.

Logan-Greene, Patricia, et al. "Protective Factors Against Aggression and Antisocial Attitudes Among Probation Youth with Childhood Adversity Histories." *Prevention Science* 24, no. 1 (2022): 161–72. https://doi.org/10.1007/s11121-022-01472-3.

Lovett, Benjamin J., and Jason M. Nelson. "Systematic Review: Educational Accommodations for Children and Adolescents with Attention-Deficit/ Hyperactivity Disorder." *Journal of the American Academy of Child and Adolescent Psychiatry*. S0890-8567(20)31333-2 (2020). https://doi.org/10.1016/j.jaac.2020.07.891.

Loy, Jik H., et al. "Atypical Antipsychotics for Disruptive Behaviour Disorders in Children and Youths." *Cochrane Database of Systematic Reviews* 2017, no. 8 (2017). https://doi.org/10.1002/14651858.cd008559.pub3.

Maenner, Matthew J., et al. "Prevalence and Characteristics of Autism Spectrum Disorder Among Children Aged 8 Years—Autism and Developmental

Disabilities Monitoring Network, 11 Sites, United States, 2020." *MMWR. Surveillance Summaries* 72, no. 2 (2023): 1–14. https://doi.org/10.15585/ mmwr.ss7202a1.

Maïano, Christophe, et al. "Prevalence of School Bullying Among Youth with Autism Spectrum Disorders: A Systematic Review and Meta-Analysis." *Autism Research* 9, no. 6 (2015): 601–15. https://doi.org/10.1002/aur.1568.

Markham, Laura. *Peaceful Parent, Happy Kids: How to Stop Yelling and Start Connecting.* New York: Perigee Book, 2012.

Marraccini, Marisa E., and Zoe M. F. Brier. "School Connectedness and Suicidal Thoughts and Behaviors: A Systematic Meta-Analysis." *School Psychology Quarterly* (March 2017). doi: 10.1037/spq0000192.

Martin, Christina Gamache, et al. "The Role of Caregiver Psychopathology in the Treatment of Childhood Trauma with Trauma-Focused Cognitive Behavioral Therapy: A Systematic Review." *Clinical Child and Family Psychology Review* 22, no. 3 (2019): 273–89. https://doi.org/10.1007/s10567 -019-00290-4.

Matheis, Maya, et al. "Factors Related to Parental Age of First Concern in Toddlers with Autism Spectrum Disorder." *Developmental Neurorehabilitation* 20, no. 4 (2016): 228–35. https://doi.org/10.1080/17518423.2016.1211186.

McLaughlin, Katie, et al. "Trauma Exposure and Posttraumatic Stress Disorder in a National Sample of Adolescents." *Journal of the American Academy of Child & Adolescent Psychiatry* 52, no. 8 (2013): 815–30. https://doi.org/doi .org/10.1016/j.jaac.2013.05.011.

Memarzia, Jessica, Jack Walker, and Richard Meiser-Stedman. "Psychological Peritraumatic Risk Factors for Post-Traumatic Stress Disorder in Children and Adolescents: A Meta-Analytic Review." *Journal of Affective Disorders* 282 (2021): 1036–47. https://doi.org/10.1016/j.jad.2021.01.016.

Mental Health: A Report of the Surgeon General (1999).

Miranda, Robert, and Hayley Treloar. "Emerging Pharmacologic Treatments for Adolescent Substance Use: Challenges and New Directions." *Current Addiction Reports* 3, no. 2 (2016): 145–56. https://doi.org/10.1007/s40429 -016-0098-7.

Miranda-Mendizabal, Andrea, et al. "Gender Differences in Suicidal Behavior in Adolescents and Young Adults: Systematic Review and Meta-Analysis of Longitudinal Studies." *International Journal of Public Health* (March 2019). doi: 10.1007/s00038-018-1196-1.

Modabbernia, Amirhossein, Eva Velthorst, and Abraham Reichenberg. "Environmental Risk Factors for Autism: An Evidence-Based Review of Systematic Reviews and Meta-Analyses." *Molecular Autism* 8, no. 1 (2017). https://doi.org/10.1186/s13229-017-0121-4.

Moncrieff, Joanna, et al. "The Serotonin Theory of Depression: A Systematic Umbrella Review of the Evidence." *Molecular Psychiatry* (2022). doi:10.1038/s41380-022-01661-0.

Morales, Angelica M., et al. "Identifying Early Risk Factors for Addiction Later in Life: A Review of Prospective Longitudinal Studies." *Current Addiction Reports* 7, no. 1 (2019): 89–98. https://doi.org/10.1007/s40429-019-00282-y.

Moreno-Alcázar, Ana, et al. "Efficacy of Eye Movement Desensitization and Reprocessing in Children and Adolescent with Post-Traumatic Stress Disorder: A Meta-Analysis of Randomized Controlled Trials." *Frontiers in Psychology* 8 (2017).

Morgan, Paul L., et al. "Racial and Ethnic Disparities in ADHD Diagnosis from Kindergarten to Eighth Grade." *Pediatrics* 132, no. 1 (2013): 85–93. https://doi.org/10.1542/peds.2012-2390.

Morina, Nexhmedin, Rachel Koerssen, and Thomas V. Pollet. "Interventions for Children and Adolescents with Posttraumatic Stress Disorder: A Meta-Analysis of Comparative Outcome Studies." *Clinical Psychology Review* 47 (2016): 41–54. https://doi.org/10.1016/j.cpr.2016.05.006.

Morken, Ida S., et al. "Explaining the Female Preponderance in Adolescent Depression—A Four-Wave Cohort Study." *Research on Child and Adolescent Psychopathology* 51, no. 6 (2023): 859–69. https://doi.org/10.1007/s10802-023-01031-6.

Mufson, Laura H., et al. *Interpersonal Psychotherapy for Depressed Adolescents* (2nd ed.). New York: Guilford Press, 2004.

Mullins, Mary Frances. "Cannabis Dabbing." *Nursing* 51, no. 5 (2021): 46–50. https://doi.org/10.1097/01.nurse.0000743108.72528.d8.

Mulraney, Melissa, et al. "Collaborative and Proactive Solutions Compared with Usual Care to Treat Irritability in Children and Adolescents: A Pilot Randomized Controlled Trial." *Clinical Psychologist* 26, no. 2 (2022): 231–39. https://doi.org/10.1080/13284207.2022.2041983.

"Multiple Cause of Death, 1999–2020 Request." Centers for Disease Control and Prevention. Accessed June 24, 2023. http://wonder.cdc.gov/mcd-icd10.html.

Murrihy, Rachael C., et al. "Community-Delivered Collaborative and Proactive Solutions and Parent Management Training for Oppositional Youth: A Randomized Trial." *Behavior Therapy* 54, no. 2 (2023): 400–417. https://doi.org/10.1016/j.beth.2022.10.005.

National Child Traumatic Stress Network. "Complex Trauma," n.d. https://www.nctsn.org/what-is-child-trauma/trauma-types/complex-trauma.

National Child Traumatic Stress Network. "Dissociation and PTSD," n.d. https://www.nctsn.org/what-is-child-trauma/trauma-types/complex-trauma.

Navarro, Raúl, et al. "Families, Parenting and Aggressive Preschoolers: A Scoping Review of Studies Examining Family Variables Related to Preschool

Bibliography

Aggression." *International Journal of Environmental Research and Public Health* 19, no. 23 (2022): 15556. https://doi.org/10.3390/ijerph192315556.

Nawi, Azmawati Mohammed, et al. "Risk and Protective Factors of Drug Abuse Among Adolescents: A Systematic Review." *BMC Public Health* 21, no. 1 (2021). https://doi.org/10.1186/s12889-021-11906-2.

Neale, Benjamin M., et al. "Meta-Analysis of Genome-Wide Association Studies of Attention-Deficit/Hyperactivity Disorder." *Journal of the American Academy of Child and Adolescent Psychiatry* 49, no. 9 (2010): 884–97. https://doi.org/10.1016/j.jaac.2010.06.008.

Ng, Michelle, et al. "Environmental Factors Associated with Autism Spectrum Disorder: A Scoping Review for the Years 2003–2013." *Health Promotion and Chronic Disease Prevention in Canada* 37, no. 1 (2017): 1–23. https://doi.org/10.24095/hpcdp.37.1.01.

Nicotra, Cassandra M., and Jeffrey R. Strawn. "Advances in Pharmacotherapy for Pediatric Anxiety Disorders." *Child and Adolescent Psychiatric Clinics of North America* 32, no. 3 (2023): 573–87. doi:10.1016/j.chc.2023.02.006.

Novo Navarro, Patricia, et al. "25 Años de Eye Movement Desensitization and Reprocessing: Protocolo de Aplicación, Hipótesis de Funcionamiento y Revisión Sistemática de Su Eficacia En El Trastorno Por Estrés Postraumático." *Revista de Psiquiatría y Salud Mental* 11, no. 2 (2018): 101–14. https://doi.org/10.1016/j.rpsm.2015.12.002.

Nowell, S., et al. "Augmentative & Alternative Communication." AFIRM, 2022. https://afirm.fpg.unc.edu/augmentative-alternative-communication.

Olfson, Mark, Steven Marcus, and George Wan. "Stimulant Dosing for Children with ADHD: A Medical Claims Analysis." *Journal of the American Academy of Child & Adolescent Psychiatry* 48, no. 1 (2009): 51–59. https://doi.org/10.1097/CHI.0b013e31818b1c8f.

Oono, Inalegwu P., Emma J. Honey, and Helen McConachie. "Parent-Mediated Early Intervention for Young Children with Autism Spectrum Disorders (ASD)." *Cochrane Database of Systematic Reviews* 4 (2013). https://doi.org/10.1002/14651858.cd009774.pub2.

Owens, Elizabeth, and Lily Hechtman. "The Berkeley Girls with ADHD Longitudinal Study." In *Attention Deficit Hyperactivity Disorder: Adult Outcome and Its Predictors*. New York: Oxford University Press, 2017, 179–229.

Perra, Oliver, Amy L. Paine, and Dale F. Hay. "Continuity and Change in Anger and Aggressiveness from Infancy to Childhood: The Protective Effects of Positive Parenting." *Development and Psychopathology* 33, no. 3 (2020): 937–56. https://doi.org/10.1017/s0954579420000243.

Perrin, Sean, Patrick Smith, and William Yule. "Practitioner Review: The Assessment and Treatment of Post-Traumatic Stress Disorder in Children and Adolescents." *Journal of Child Psychology and Psychiatry and Allied Disciplines* 41, no. 3 (2000): 277–89.

Phelan, Thomas W. *1-2-3 Magic: Effective Discipline for Children 2–12.* Naperville, IL: Sourcebooks, 2016.

Platt, Jonathan M., et al. "Is the US Gender Gap in Depression Changing Over Time? A Meta-Regression." *American Journal of Epidemiology* 190, no. 7 (2021): 1190–1206. https://doi.org/10.1093/aje/kwab002.

Punja, Salima, et al. "Amphetamines for Attention Deficit Hyperactivity Disorder (ADHD) in Children and Adolescents." *Cochrane Database of Systematic Reviews* 2 (2016): 471–77. https://doi.org/10.1177/1087054715605915.

Quagliato, Laiana A., Ursula M. A. de Matos, and Antonio E. Nardi. "Lifetime Psychopathology in the Offspring of Parents with Anxiety Disorders: A Systematic Review." *Journal of Affective Disorders* 319 (2022): 618–26. doi:10.1016/j.jad.2022.09.049.

Quigley, Jody, Susan Rasmussen, and John McAlaney. "The Social Norms of Suicidal and Self-Harming Behaviors in Scottish Adolescents." *International Journal of Environmental Research and Public Health* (2017), http://dx.doi.ord/10.3390/ijerph14030307.

Ramsey, Emily, et al. "Autism Spectrum Disorder Prevalence Rates in the United States: Methodologies, Challenges, and Implications for Individual States." *Journal of Developmental and Physical Disabilities* 28, no. 1 (2016): 803–20. https://doi.org/10.1007/s10882-016-9510-4.

Ray, Dee C. *Advanced Play Therapy: Essential Conditions, Knowledge, and Skills for Child Practice.* New York: Routledge, Taylor & Francis Group, 2021.

Reamer, Frederic G., and Deborah H. Siegel. *Teens in Crisis: How the Industry Serving Struggling Teens Helps and Hurts Our Kids.* New York: Columbia University Press, 2008.

Reichow, Brian. "Overview of Meta-Analyses on Early Intensive Behavioral Intervention for Young Children with Autism Spectrum Disorders." *Journal of Autism and Developmental Disorders* 42 (2012): 512–20. https://doi.org/10.1007/s10803-011-1218-9.

Remes, Olivia, et al. "A Systematic Review of Reviews on the Prevalence of Anxiety Disorders in Adult Populations." *Brain and Behavior* 6, no. 7 (2016): e00497. doi:10-1002/brb3.497.

Risch, Neil, et al. "Familial Recurrence of Autism Spectrum Disorder: Evaluating Genetic and Environmental Contributions." *American Journal of Psychiatry* 171, no. 11 (2014): 1206–13. https://doi.org/10.1176/appi.ajp.2014.13101359.

Riva, Anna, et al. "Eating Disorders in Children and Adolescent Males: A Peculiar Psychopathological Profile." *International Journal of Environmental*

Research and Public Health 19, no. 18 (2022): 11449. https://doi.org/10.3390/ijerph191811449.

Rosa-Alcázar, Ángel, et al. "Cognitive-Behavioral Therapy and Anxiety and Depression Level in Pediatric Obsessive-Compulsive Disorder: A Systematic Review and Meta-Analysis." *Psicothema* 34, no. 3 (2022): 353–64. doi:10.7334/psicothema2021.478.

Rosenberg, Rebecca E., et al. "Factors Affecting Age at Initial Autism Spectrum Disorder Diagnosis in a National Survey." *Autism Research and Treatment*, 2011, 1–11. https://doi.org/10.1155/2011/874619.

Rossignol, D. A., S. J. Genuis, and R. E. Frye. "Environmental Toxicants and Autism Spectrum Disorders: A Systematic Review." *Translational Psychiatry* 4, no. 2 (2014). https://doi.org/10.1038/tp.2014.4.

Roubinov, Danielle, et al. "Intergenerational Transmission of Maternal Childhood Adversity and Depression on Children's Internalizing Problems." *Journal of Affective Disorders* 308 (2022), 205–12.

Rowe, Richard, et al. "Developmental Pathways in Oppositional Defiant Disorder and Conduct Disorder." *Journal of Abnormal Psychology* 119, no. 4 (2010): 726–38. https://doi.org/10.1037/a0020798.

Russell, Mark C., and Francine Shapiro. *Eye Movement Desensitization and Reprocessing (EMDR) Therapy*. Washington, DC: American Psychological Association, 2022.

Sam, A., and AFIRM Team. "Prompting." AFIRM, 2015. http://afirm.fpg.unc.edu/prompting.

Sam, A., and AFIRM Team. "Social Narratives." AFIRM, 2015. http://afirm.fpg.unc.edu/social-narratives.

Sam, A., and AFIRM Team. "Visual Supports." AFIRM, 2015. http://afirm.fpg.unc.edu/visual-supports.

Sam, A., et al. "Selecting an Evidence-Based Practice." AFIRM, 2022. https://afirm.fpg.unc.edu/selecting-evidence-based-practice.

Sarvet, Aaron L., et al. "Medical Marijuana Laws and Adolescent Marijuana Use in the United States: A Systematic Review and Meta-Analysis." *Addiction* 113, no. 6 (2018): 1003–16. https://doi.org/10.1111/add.14136.

Schaeffer, Cindy M., et al. "A Smartphone App for Parental Management of Adolescent Conduct Problems: Randomized Clinical Trial of iKinnect." *Journal of Clinical Child and Adolescent Psychology* (2022): 1–15.

Schubart, Jane R., Fabian Camacho, and Douglas Leslie. "Psychotropic Medication Trends Among Children and Adolescents with Autism Spectrum Disorder in the Medicaid Program." *Autism: The International Journal of Research and Practice* 18, no. 6 (2014): 631–37. https://doi.org/10.1177/1362361313497537.

Scull, Andrew. *Desperate Remedies: Psychiatry's Turbulent Quest to Cure Mental Illness*. Cambridge, MA: Belknap Press of Harvard University Press, 2022.

Seok, Ji-Woo, et al. "Psychopharmacological Treatment of Disruptive Behavior in Youths: Systematic Review and Network Meta-Analysis." *Scientific Reports* 13, no. 1 (2023). https://doi.org/10.1038/s41598-023-33979-2.

Serafini, Gianluca, et al. "Life Adversities and Suicidal Behavior in Young Individuals: A Systematic Review." *European Child and Adolescent Psychiatry* (2015). doi: 10.1007/s00787-015-0760-y.

"Sexuality for All Abilities Curriculum." Mad Hatter Wellness, n.d. https://madhatterwellness.com/product/curriculum/%20.

Shaw, Monica, et al. "A Systematic Review and Analysis of Long-Term Outcomes in Attention Deficit Hyperactivity Disorder: Effects of Treatment and Non-Treatment." *BMC Medicine* 10 (2012): 99. http://doi.org/10.1186/1741-7015-10-99.

Shi, Yuyan, Sharon E. Cummins, and Shu-Hong Zhu. "Medical Marijuana Availability, Price, and Product Variety, and Adolescents' Marijuana Use." *Journal of Adolescent Health* 63, no. 1 (2018): 88–93. https://doi.org/10.1016/j.jadohealth.2018.01.008.

Shore, Lori, et al. "Longitudinal Trajectories of Child and Adolescent Depressive Symptoms and Their Predictors—A Systematic Review and Meta-Analysis." *Child and Adolescent Mental Health* 23, no. 2 (2018): 107–20.

Shoval, Gal, et al. "Evaluation of Attention-Deficit/Hyperactivity Disorder Medications, Externalizing Symptoms, and Suicidality in Children." *JAMA Network Open* 4, no. 6 (2021). https://doi.org/10.1001/jamanetworkopen.2021.11342.

Sigurvinsdóttir, Anna Lilja, et al. "Effectiveness of Cognitive Behavioral Therapy (CBT) for Child and Adolescent Anxiety Disorders Across Different CBT Modalities and Comparisons: A Systematic Review and Meta-Analysis." *Nordic Journal of Psychiatry* 74, no. 3 (2020): 168–80. doi:10.1080/08039488.2019.1686653.

Solmi, Marco, et al. "Age at Onset of Mental Disorders Worldwide: Large-Scale Meta-Analysis of 192 Epidemiological Studies." *Molecular Psychiatry* 27 (2022): 281–95. https://doi.org/10.1038/s41380-021-01161-7.

Soria-Saucedo, Rene, et al. "Factors That Predict the Use of Psychotropics Among Children and Adolescents with PTSD: Evidence from Private Insurance Claims." *Psychiatric Services* 69, no. 9 (2018): 1007–14. https://doi.org/10.1176/appi.ps.201700167.

Steinbrecher, A., et al. "Supported Decision Making in Delaware." Delaware Network for Excellence in Autism, 2023. https://www.delawareautismnetwork

.org/wp-content/uploads/2023/04/SupportedDecision-MakingInDelaware
.pdf.

Stice, Eric, C. Nathan Marti, and Paul Rohde. "Prevalence, Incidence, Impairment, and Course of the Proposed DSM-5 Eating Disorder Diagnoses in an 8-Year Prospective Community Study of Young Women." *Journal of Abnormal Psychology* 122, no. 2 (2013): 445–57. https://doi.org/10.1037/a0030679.

Stoddard, Joel, et al. "An Open Pilot Study of Training Hostile Interpretation Bias to Treat Disruptive Mood Dysregulation Disorder." *Journal of Child and Adolescent Psychopharmacology* 26, no. 1 (2016): 49–57. https://doi.org/10.1089/cap.2015.0100.

Sullivan, Patrick F., Michael C. Neale, and Kenneth S. Kendler. "Genetic Epidemiology of Major Depression: Review and Meta-Analysis." *American Journal of Psychiatry* 157, no. 10 (2000): 1552–62.

Sundgot-Borgen, Jorunn, and Monica Klungland Torstveit. "Prevalence of Eating Disorders in Elite Athletes Is Higher Than in the General Population." *Clinical Journal of Sport Medicine* 14, no. 1 (2004): 25–32. https://doi.org/10.1097/00042752-200401000-00005.

Swanson, James, et al. "Evidence, Interpretation, and Qualification from Multiple Reports of Long-Term Outcomes in the Multimodal Treatment Study of Children with ADHD (MTA): Part I: Executive Summary." *Journal of Attention Disorders* 12, no. 1 (2008): 4–14. https://doi.org/10.1177/1087054708319345.

Swanson, Sonja A., et al. "Prevalence and Correlates of Eating Disorders in Adolescents." *Archives of General Psychiatry* 68, no. 7 (2011): 714. https://doi.org/10.1001/archgenpsychiatry.2011.22.

Taliaferro, Lindsay A., et al. "Profiles of Risk and Protection for Violence and Bullying Perpetration Among Adolescent Boys." *Journal of School Health* 90, no. 3 (2020): 212–23. https://doi.org/10.1111/josh.12867.

Tan, Eng Joo, et al. "The Association Between Eating Disorders and Mental Health: An Umbrella Review." *Journal of Eating Disorders* 11, no. 1 (2023). https://doi.org/10.1186/s40337-022-00725-4.

Tanner-Smith, Emily E., Sandra Jo Wilson, and Mark W. Lipsey. "The Comparative Effectiveness of Outpatient Treatment for Adolescent Substance Abuse: A Meta-Analysis." *Journal of Substance Abuse Treatment* 44, no. 2 (2013): 145–58. https://doi.org/10.1016/j.jsat.2012.05.006.

Tao, Yuanmei, et al. "Comparing the Efficacy of Pharmacological and Psychological Treatment, Alone and in Combination, in Children and Adolescents with Obsessive-Compulsive Disorder: A Network Meta-Analysis." *Journal of Psychiatric Research* 148 (2022): 95–102.

Tick, Beata, et al. "Heritability of Autism Spectrum Disorders: A Meta-Analysis of Twin Studies." *Journal of Child Psychology and Psychiatry* 57, no. 5 (2016): 585–95. https://doi.org/10.1111/jcpp.12499.

Tindall, Lucy, et al. "Is Behavioural Activation Effective in the Treatment of Depression in Young People? A Systematic Review and Meta-Analysis." *Psychology and Psychotherapy: Theory, Research, Practice, Training* 90, no. 4 (March 2017): 770–96.

Toole-Anstey, Chye, Lynne Keevers, and Michelle L. Townsend. "A Systematic Review of Child to Parent Violence Interventions." *Trauma, Violence, & Abuse* 24, no. 2 (2023): 1157–71. https://doi.org/10.1177/15248380211053618.

Tormohlen, Kayla N., et al. "Changes in Prevalence of Marijuana Consumption Modes Among Colorado High School Students from 2015 to 2017." *JAMA Pediatrics* 173, no. 10 (2019): 988–89. https://doi.org/10.1001/jamapediatrics.2019.2627.

Trujillo, Carlos Andres, Diana Obando, and Angela Trujillo. "An Examination of the Association Between Early Initiation of Substance Use and Interrelated Multilevel Risk and Protective Factors Among Adolescents." *PLOS One* 14, no. 12 (2019). https://doi.org/10.1371/journal.pone.0225384.

Tse, Zoie Wai Man, et al. "School-Based Cognitive-Behavioural Therapy for Children and Adolescents with Social Anxiety Disorder and Social Anxiety Symptoms: A Systematic Review." *PLOS One* 18, no. 3 (2023): e0283329. doi:10.1371/journal.pone.0283329.

Tucker, James R. D., and Christopher W. Hobson. "A Systematic Review of Longitudinal Studies Investigating the Association Between Early Life Maternal Depression and Offspring ADHD." *Journal of Attention Disorders* 26, no. 9 (2022): 1167–86. http://doi.org/10.1177/10870547211063642.

Tung, Irene, et al. "Patterns of Comorbidity Among Girls with ADHD: A Meta-Analysis." *Pediatrics* 138, no. 4 (2016): https://doi.org/10.1542/peds.2016-0430.

Uchida, M., et al. "The Heritability of ADHD in Children of ADHD Parents: A Post-Hoc Analysis of Longitudinal Data." *Journal of Attention Disorders* 27, no. 3 (2023): 250–57. https://doi.org/10.1177/10870547221136251.

Vibkufar, Viktoria, et al. "A Systematic Review and Meta-Analysis on the Prevalence of Depression in Children and Adolescents After Exposure to Trauma." *Journal of Affective Disorders* 255 (2019): 77–89. https://doi.org/doi.org/10.1016/j.jad.2019.05.005.

Vierck, Esther, and Jeremy M. Silverman. "Brief Report: Phenotypic Differences and Their Relationship to Paternal Age and Gender in Autism Spectrum Disorder." *Journal of Autism and Developmental Disorders* 45 (2015): 1915–24. https://doi.org/10.1007/s10803-014-2346-9.

Visser, Susana N., et al. "Demographic Differences Among a National Sample of US Youth with Behavioral Disorders." *Clinical Pediatrics* 55, no. 14 (2016): 1358–62. https://doi.org/10.1177/0009922815623229.

Walter, Heather J., et al. "Clinical Practice Guideline for the Assessment and Treatment of Children and Adolescents with Major and Persistent Depressive Disorders." *Journal of the American Academy of Child & Adolescent Psychiatry* 62, no. 5 (October 2022): 479–502. https://doi.org/10.1016/j.jaac.2022.10.001.

Warner, Emily N., and Jeffrey R. Strawn. "Risk Factors for Pediatric Anxiety Disorders." *Child and Adolescent Psychiatric Clinics of North America* 32, no. 3 (2023): 485–510. https://doi.org/10.1016/j.chc.2022.10.001.

Warner, Emily N., et al. "Developmental Epidemiology of Pediatric Anxiety Disorders." *Child and Adolescent Psychiatric Clinics of North America* 32, no. 3 (2023): 511–30. doi:10.1016/j.chc.2023.02.001.

Waszczuk, Monika A., Helena M. Zavos, and Thalia C. Eley. "Why Do Depression, Conduct, and Hyperactivity Symptoms Co-Occur Across Adolescence? The Role of Stable and Dynamic Genetic and Environmental Influences." *European Child & Adolescent Psychiatry* 30, no. 7 (2021): 1013–25. https://doi.org/10.1007/s00787-020-01515-6.

Watson, Hunna J., et al. "Genetics of Eating Disorders in the Genome-Wide Era." *Psychological Medicine* 51, no. 13 (2021): 2287–97. https://doi.org/10.1017/s0033291720005474.

Waxmonsky, James G., et al. "A Commercial Insurance Claims Analysis of Correlates of Behavioral Therapy Use Among Children with ADHD." *Psychiatric Services* 70, no. 12 (2019): 1116–22. https://doi.org/10.1176/appi.ps.201800473.

Weinberger, A. H., et al. "Trends in Depression Prevalence in the USA from 2005 to 2015: Widening Disparities in Vulnerable Groups." *Psychological Medicine* 48, no. 8 (2018): 1308–15. doi: 10.1017/S0033291717002781.

Wesemann, Daniel. "Pharmacological Treatment for Pediatric Anxiety Disorders." *Journal of Psychosocial Nursing and Mental Health Services* 60, no. 9 (2022): 6–9. doi:10.3928/02793695-20220809-04.

Whitney, Daniel G., and Mark D. Peterson. "US National and State-Level Prevalence of Mental Health Disorders and Disparities of Mental Health Care Use in Children." *JAMA Pediatrics* 173, no. 4 (2019): 389–91. https://doi.org/10.1001/jamapediatrics.2018.5399.

Wilens, Timothy E., et al. "The Impact of Pharmacotherapy of Childhood-Onset Psychiatric Disorders on the Development of Substance Use Disorders." *Journal of Child and Adolescent Psychopharmacology* 32, no. 4 (2022): 200–214. https://doi.org/10.1089/cap.2022.0016.

Winters, Drew E., et al. "Improvements in Irritability with Open-Label Methylphenidate Treatment in Youth with Comorbid Attention Deficit/

Hyperactivity Disorder and Disruptive Mood Dysregulation Disorder." *Journal of Child and Adolescent Psychopharmacology* 28, no. 5 (2018): 298–305. https://doi.org/10.1089/cap.2017.0124.

Witt, Katrina, et al. "Psychosocial Interventions for People Who Self-Harm: Methodological Issues Involved with Trials to Evaluate Effectiveness." *Archives of Suicide Research* (2019): 1–81. doi: 10.1080/13811118.2019.1592043.

Wolraich, Mark L., et al. "Clinical Practice Guideline for the Diagnosis, Evaluation, and Treatment of Attention-Deficit/Hyperactivity Disorder in Children and Adolescents." *Pediatrics* 144, no. 4 (2019): e20192528. https://doi.org/10.1542/peds.2019-2528.

Woolgar, Francesca, et al. "Systematic Review and Meta-Analysis: Prevalence of Posttraumatic Stress Disorder in Trauma-Exposed Preschool-Aged Children." *Journal of the American Academy of Child and Adolescent Psychiatry* 61, no. 3 (2022): 366–77. https://doi.org/doi.org/10.1016/j.jaac.2021.05.026.

Wüstner, Anne, et al. "Risk and Protective Factors for the Development of ADHD Symptoms in Children and Adolescents: Results of the Longitudinal BELLA Study." *PLOS One* 14, no. 3 (2019): https://doi.org/10.1371/journal.pone.0214412.

Wymbs, Brian T., et al. "Early Adolescent Substance Use as a Risk Factor for Developing Conduct Disorder and Depression Symptoms." *Journal of Studies on Alcohol and Drugs* 75, no. 2 (2014): 279–89. https://doi.org/10.15288/jsad.2014.75.279.

Xiang, Yajie, et al. "Comparative Short-Term Efficacy and Acceptability of a Combination of Pharmacotherapy and Psychotherapy for Depressive Disorder in Children and Adolescents: A Systematic Review and Meta-Analysis." *BMC Psychiatry* 22, no. 1 (February 2022). https://doi.org/10.1186/s12888-022-03760-2.

Xie, Pingxing, et al. "Interactive Effect of Stressful Life Events and the Serotonin Transporter 5-HTTLPR Genotype on Posttraumatic Stress Disorder Diagnosis in 2 Independent Populations." *Archives of General Psychiatry* 66, no. 11 (2009): 1201. https://doi.org/10.1001/archgenpsychiatry.2009.153.

Yager, Joel, et al. "Guideline Watch (August 2012): Practice Guideline for the Treatment of Patients with Eating Disorders, 3rd Edition." *FOCUS* 12, no. 4 (2014): 416–31. https://doi.org/10.1176/appi.focus.120404.

Yohros, Alexis. "Examining the Relationship Between Adverse Childhood Experiences and Juvenile Recidivism: A Systematic Review and Meta-Analysis." *Trauma, Violence, & Abuse* 24, no. 3 (2023): 1640–55. https://doi.org/10.1177/15248380211073846.

Youth Risk Behavior Survey—Centers for Disease Control and Prevention, n.d. https://www.cdc.gov/healthyyouth/data/yrbs/pdf/YRBS_Data-Summary-Trends_Report2023_508.pdf?mc_cid=d112968ed9&mc_eid=80b51934b7.

Yu, Qiongru, et al. "Roads Diverged: Developmental Trajectories of Irritability from Toddlerhood through Adolescence." *Journal of the American Academy of Child and Adolescent Psychiatry* 62, no. 4 (2023): 457–71. https://doi.org/10.1016/j.jaac.2022.07.849.

Resources

CHAPTER 1: ATTENTION-DEFICIT HYPERACTIVITY DISORDER

Barkley, Russell. *Taking Charge of ADHD: The Authoritative Guide for Parents*, 4th ed., Guilford Publications, 2020.

https://www.russellbarkley.org

https://www.youtube.com/watch?v=zUA6esXOZcs

https://www.youtube.com/watch?v=SCAGc-rkIfo

Children and Adults with Attention-Deficit and Hyperactivity Disorder (CHADD): https://chadd.org (Note: About a million dollars a funding a year, or a third of CHADD's funding, comes from pharmaceutical companies.) They have a lot of resources on this website, including support groups in your area.

GoodRx: a free app that tells you where the medication is at nearby drugstores and how much it costs at each.

Social media resources and forums for parents of children with ADHD: https://www.friendshipcircle.org/blog/2014/02/24/30-addadhd-resources-you-should-follow-on-social-media/.

CHAPTER 2: AUTISM SPECTRUM DISORDERS

Brill, S., and M. Kenney. *The Transgender Teen: A Handbook for Parents and Professionals Supporting Transgender and Non-Binary Teens.* San Francisco: Cleis Press, 2016.

Ehrensaft, Diane, and Edgardo Menvielle. *Gender Born, Gender Made: Raising Healthy Gender-Nonconforming Children.* New York: Experiment, 2011.

Ehrensaft, Diane, and Norman Spack. *The Gender Creative Child: Pathways for Nurturing and Supporting Children Who Live Outside Gender Boxes.* Mulgrave, Australia: Simon & Schuster Australia, 2017.

Lev, Arlene Istar, and Andrew R. Gottlieb. *Families in Transition: Parenting Gender Diverse Children, Adolescents, and Young Adults.* New York: Harrington Park Press, 2019.

Sheryl, K., and S. Brill. *The Transgender Child: A Handbook for Families and Professionals.* San Francisco: Cleis Press, 2008.

CHAPTER 3: DEPRESSIVE DISORDERS, SELF-HARM, AND SUICIDALITY

For finding a qualified therapist: Anxiety and Depression Associates of America: https://members.adaa.org/page/FATMain

For finding a list of interpersonal therapy providers: Here is the directory of trained IPT therapists: https://iptinstitute.com/ipt-directory/

Adolescent Coping with Depression course freely downloadable to therapists: https://research.kpchr.org/Research/Research-Areas/Mental-Health/Youth -Depression-Programs#Downloads

Resources for LGBTQ youth and their parents:

PFLAG is a wealth of educational resources and potential local support groups. https://pflag.org/find-resources/

Family Acceptance Project, https://familyproject.sfsu.edu

CHAPTER 4: ANXIETY AND OBSESSIVE-COMPULSIVE DISORDER

Lebowitz, Eli R.. *Breaking Free of Child Anxiety and OCD: A Scientifically Proven Program for Parents.* New York: Oxford University Press, 2021.

Rapee, Ronald M., Ann Wignall, Susan Spence, Vanessa Cobham, and Heidi
  J. Lyneham. *Helping Your Anxious Child: A Step-by-Step Guide for Parents.*
  Oakland, CA: New Harbinger Publications, Inc., 2022.
Picture books about anxiety to read to your preschooler/early elementary age
  child: https://bookriot.com/picture-books-about-anxiety
To find qualified therapists:
  • https://www.med.upenn.edu/ctsa/Find_an_Ex/RP_Therapist.html
  • International OCD Foundation: https://iocdf.org/find-help/
  • Anxiety and Depression Associates of America: https://members
    .adaa.org/page/FATMain

CHAPTER 5: EATING DISORDERS

https://www.nationaleatingdisorders.org/screening-tool.
https://www.feast-ed.org/feast-30-days/.

CHAPTER 6: POST-TRAUMATIC STRESS DISORDER

"Home–Child-Parent Psychotherapy." Child-Parent Psychotherapy, May 22,
  2023. https://childparentpsychotherapy.com/.
Naish, Sarah. *The A-Z of Therapeutic Parenting: Strategies and Solutions.*
  London: Jessica Kingsley Publishing, 2018.
The National Child Traumatic Stress Network. Accessed July 28, 2023. https:
  //www.nctsn.org/.

CHAPTER 7: OPPOSITIONAL DEFIANT AND DISRUPTIVE MOOD DYSREGULATION DISORDERS

"30 Essential Ideas You Should Know About ADHD, 1A Intro, Chronic
  Developmental Disability." YouTube, 2014. https://www.youtube.com/
  watch?v=BzhbAK1pdPM.
Barkley, Russell A., and C. Benton. *Your Defiant Child. Eight Steps to Better
  Behavior*, 2nd ed. New York: Guilford Press, 2013.

Cline, Foster, and Jim Fay. *Parenting with Love and Logic: Teaching Children Responsibility*. 3rd ed. Colorado Springs, CO: NavPress Publishing Group, 2020.

Greene, Ross W. *The Explosive Child: A New Approach for Understanding and Parenting Easily Frustrated, Chronically Inflexible Children*. New York: Harper, 2021.

Kazdin, Alan E. *The Kazdin Method for Parenting the Defiant Child: With No Pills, No Therapy, No Contest of Wills*. Boston: Houghton Mifflin Harcourt, 2009.

Markham, Lauren. *Peaceful Parent, Happy Kids: How to Stop Yelling and Start Connecting*. New York: Perigee Book, 2012.

Phelan, Thomas W. *1-2-3 Magic: Effective Discipline for Children 2–12*. Glen Ellyn, IL: Parent Magic, 2004.

Steiner, Hans, and Lisa Remsing. Odd—AACAP. Accessed July 12, 2023. https://www.aacap.org/App_Themes/AACAP/docs/resource_centers/odd/odd_resource_center_odd_guide.pdf.

Wexelblatt, Ryan. "Effective Solutions for Parents of Children with ADHD." ADHD Dude, n.d., https://adhddude.com/.

CHAPTER 8: ADOLESCENT CONDUCT AND SUBSTANCE USE DISORDERS

Barkley, Russell A., and Arthur Robin. *Your Defiant Teen. 10 Steps to Resolve Conflict and Rebuild Your Relationship*. New York: Guilford Press, 2014.
https://www.samhsa.gov/talk-they-hear-you/parent-resources/why-you-should-talk-your-child.

CHAPTER 9: ACCESSING SERVICES AND NAVIGATING THE SYSTEM

The Centers for Disease Control (CDC) offers a comprehensive, step-by-step process on how to access screening and assessment for your child before they enter school, which can be found at this link: https://www.cdc.gov/ncbddd/actearly/concerned.html.

Questions to ask if you are considering hiring an educational advocate: https://www.understood.org/en/articles/how-to-find-a-special-education-advocate.

Therapeutic boarding schools: The National Association of Therapeutic Schools and Programs' website: https://natsap.org/.

A list of residential treatment programs by state (not necessarily complete): https://childresidentialtreatment.com/wilderness-therapy-programs/.

A list of programs for "troubled teens": https://www.eprogramsearch.com.

CHAPTER 10: PARENTING INTERVENTIONS

Couples Therapy and Self-Help

Christensen, Andrew, Brian D. Doss, and Neil S. Jacobson. *Reconcilable Differences: Rebuild Your Relationship by Rediscovering the Partner You Love—Without Losing Yourself.* New York: Guilford Press, 2014.

Emotionally focused couples therapy: https://iceeft.com/what-is-eft/.

Gottman Couples Institute: https://www.gottman.com/couples/find-a-therapist/.

Gottman, John Mordechai, and Nan Silver. *The Seven Principles for Making Marriage Work: A Practical Guide from the Country's Foremost Relationship Expert.* New York: Harmony Books, 2015.

Hendrix, Harville, and Helen Hunt. *Getting the Love You Want: A Guide for Couples.* New York: Henry Holt & Company, 2022.

Imago therapy: https://harvilleandhelen.com/#.

Integrative Behavioral Couples therapy: https://ibct.psych.ucla.edu/.

Johnson, Sue. *The Hold Me Tight Workbook: A Couples Guide for a Lifetime of Love.* New York: Little, Brown Spark, 2022.

Self-Help Alternatives for Substance Use Disorders

S.M.A.R.T. Recovery (based on principles of motivational interviewing and Cognitive Behavior Therapy: http://www.smartrecovery.org/)

- Women for Sobriety (a self-help group developed specifically for women, http://www.womenforsobriety.org/)
- HAMS (Harm Reduction), https://hams.cc/
- Moderation Management, https://moderation.org/
- LifeRing Secular Recovery, https://lifering.org/lifering-recovery-menu/
- Secular Organizations for Sobriety (SOS), http://www.sossobriety.org/

Free Support

National Alliance on Mental Illness (NAMI): https:www.nami.org.

Parenting support groups: https://www.parentshelpingparents.org/virtual
-support-groups.

Family Connections: https://www.borderlinepersonalitydisorder.org/family
-connections/.

Note that despite the reference to borderline personality disorder in this link,
this family program is for all caregivers of children who are emotionally
dysregulated and difficult to manage as a result.

Index

Page references for figures are italicized.

disorders, 78; for depressive disorders, 63; for eating disorders, 88–89; for obsessive-compulsive disorder (OCD), 78

separation disorder, 65. *See also* anxiety disorders

services, 145–58, 159–63. *See also* parenting interventions; transportation assistance

social anxiety disorder, 65. *See also* anxiety disorders

stress and trauma related disorders. *See* post–traumatic stress disorder (PTSD)

substance use disorders (SUD), 129–42; contributing factors, 130–35; interventions, 136–39; medication, 141–42; parenting, 135–36; risk and protecting

factors, 130–35; symptoms, 129; violence and juvenile justice involvement, 139–41. *See also* school system, navigating the; treatment settings

substance use disorders (SUB) as a comorbid diagnosis. *See* attention-deficit hyperactivity disorder (ADHD); conduct disorder

transportation assistance, 150–51

treatment settings: education consultants, 150; home visiting, 146–47; hospitalization, 86, 146–48; partial hospitalization, 86, 146; residential treatment centers (RTCs), 86, 148; wilderness programs, 149–50

About the Author

Jacqueline Corcoran lives in the Virginia suburbs of Washington, DC, with her family. She is a tenured professor at the University of Pennsylvania School of Social Policy and Practice. She teaches child and adolescent mental health, clinical assessment, cognitive behavioral therapy, and research to graduate students in social work. She is also the director of the Clinical Doctorate Program.

Dr. Corcoran has written twenty books and over one hundred articles and book chapters, including *Child and Adolescent Mental Health in Social Work* (2023, Oxford University Press); *Clinical Assessment and Diagnosis in Social Work Practice* (4th edition, 2022, Oxford University Press); *Mental Health in Social Work: A Casebook on Diagnosis and Strengths-Based Assessment* (3rd edition, 2019, Pearson Publishing); and *Living with Mental Disorder: Insights from Qualitative Research* (2016, Routledge).

Dr. Corcoran has been a clinical social worker for thirty years, and much of that time has been with children and families—at Child Protective Services, Victim Services, a community monitoring program for justice-involved youth, college counseling, and outpatient mental health. From these professional as well as lived experiences, she has gained much appreciation, understanding, and insight into the turmoil of families when children have mental health diagnoses and hopes to impart key information, practical wisdom, and the latest evidence-backed strategies in *Your Child's Mental Health Diagnosis: A Comprehensive and Compassionate Guide for Parents.*